MURDER ON MY MIND

A MEMOIR OF MENOPAUSE

DANA GOLDSTEIN

ALSO BY DANA GOLDSTEIN

The Girl in the Gold Bikini: My turbulent journey through food and family

Reader reviews from Amazon

"This is an incredibly entertaining book. It's a brave and raw story. Highly recommend this honest and relatable story. Easy to read and will keeps you engaged throughout!"

"An amazing story, that gripped me end to end."

"At times I was gasping in disbelief, only to start laughing or crying a minute later as I realized that what I was reading was so true not only for the amazingly honest and open author but for myself as well."

"I couldn't put the book down, but didn't want the reading of it to be over too quickly."

Published by Digital Shoebox Inc

Author page: www.danagoldstein.ca

Cover design by Dina Ferreira Stoddard www.klutchphotography.com

Image credits: Janet Pliszka (Author photo) www.visualhues.com

ISBN (paperback): 978-1-7751438-3-3

ISBN (e-book): 978-1-7751438-4-0

DISCLAIMER

I am not a medical doctor and, as such, nothing in this book should be considered medical advice. The content within these pages is intended to be anecdotal and is reflective only of my own experiences. Please consult with your doctor for your own medical questions and concerns. Not everyone is equipped to manage this insanity on their own, as I did. As a writer, I am inclined to suffer for my art so I can better share the story. In hindsight, a little serotonin boost from antidepressants might have been wise.

Dedicated to my uterus and to the three men who had a vested interest in it: Jeff, Mason, and Westin. I couldn't have done any of this without you.

CONTENTS

NOT YOUR MOTHER'S PERIMENOPAUSE

When my mother moved into assisted living, I began the arduous task of cleaning out the condo where she had lived for more than 30 years. It had been my home, too, throughout my university years. When I walked into the condo, after not being in that space for more than 15 years, I felt sad. Her whole life was about to be packed into boxes and thrown away. I tried to separate myself from the emotional reaction and focus on cleaning the mess she left behind. In the next second, I was angry, then overwhelmed, and then I had to pee. As I emptied my bladder, I awkwardly leaned forward and to the left to open the cabinet under the sink. Underneath was a single roll of toilet paper, a scrub brush, and a paper can of Comet scouring powder, its metal top so rusted out I couldn't tell where the original scattering holes were. I laughed, knowing two things had happened here.

1. My mother kept everything until the last drop was used, regardless of how many decades had passed; and

2. This was where I got my obsessive need to squeeze and roll the toothpaste tighter than a joint to get every drop.

My mother saved everything, "just in case," she used to say. She had the plastic-wrapped cups from a Howard Johnson hotel we stayed in for a few days in the summer of 1983. In the under-sink cabinet in the master bathroom, I found an unreasonable number of makeup travel bags, all clearly a "gift with purchase." The amount of stuff I was going to have throw out and sift through was astounding.

But among all the garbage, there were some gems.

Going through the drawers in her master bedroom night tables was like going back in time. Each table had two drawers, all equally packed with paper. In one drawer, I found a yellow, legal-sized envelope with the court transcript from my parents' divorce in 1981. A little further down into the pile, I came across a notebook where she chronicled the guests at their wedding in 1965, listing the gift that was given, or indicating in bold letters NO GIFT. In another drawer, I was thrilled to find she kept my letter of recommendation for a journalism fellowship. But when I flipped it over, my heart sank. She'd written a list of painters and their phone numbers on it.

Among the clutter, I found a letter penned in 1989 by 19-year-old me. I cringed as I read it for the first time in decades. The letter was addressed "To Whom it May Concern" and in it I wrote of the alarming actions of my mother, all cloaked in juvenile humour so I wouldn't be in too much trouble.

"Please save me," I wrote, "should she completely lose her mind. I have so much left to give this world."

I complained about her irrational behaviour (yelling at me for coming home late from my job) and her inability to remember anything about her own daughter (like that fact that I have *never* liked onions. Like, ever). I wrote a paragraph about how she was scaring off her friends, attacking them for some perceived slight and then trying to make me feel guilty for going out with my own friends and not inviting her. I begged for anyone to help, to make my suffering (and hers) short-lived, and to spare me from prolonged exposure to her crazy.

I can't remember what prompted me to write the letter, but I know I wrote it as a means of helping my mother identify what I saw was happening. I made reference in the letter to "The Change." At 19, I was able to figure out that my mother was in the midst of her menopausal journey, that her unreasonable and volatile behaviour was something she couldn't control and wouldn't acknowledge.

The letter wasn't particularly well-written, nor was the humour anything more than juvenile. What I had here, I realized, was evidence of my mother's own struggle with menopausal mood swings around the time she was 43.

While I started my perimenopause earlier than she did, I paused to consider that maybe the letter could give me some idea of what I might expect for my own journey. In a moment of denial, I chucked the letter into the bag of paperwork destined for the shredder.

Perimenopause lasts years, while menopause only lasts a day — the day that marks one year without a period. Postmenopause takes over from there, but the ride isn't immediately over.

My mother had refused to acknowledge what she was going through. I, on the other hand, was going to fully embrace the crazy and sometimes even have fun with it, as you'll see in the pages of this book. I wasn't going to make this a hell for my kids like my mother made it for me. Ah, the lies we tell ourselves.

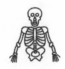

ONE

DIAGNOSIS

I sat on the edge of the table in the doctor's office, swinging my legs like a toddler, waiting for the results of multiple tests. This was only my second visit with this doctor, and I wasn't sure if I liked her. She was Russian, but that isn't what made me uncomfortable. I know how to handle Russian women. I had grown up with strong and smart Russian women all around me. I learned at an early age you don't mess with women who spent hours standing in line in the middle of a Moscow winter waiting for a loaf of bread and some eggs. They fear nothing. And they don't take your shit.

This doctor had the same no-nonsense approach. She was clinical and so judgmental with a serious deficiency in bedside manner. On my first visit, she performed my annual Pap smear, and she grunted as she manipulated the speculum, like she was trying to pry open a jar of pickles.

"You have regular sex, hmmm," she muttered from between my thighs at that checkup.

I didn't know if she was asking or observing. I opted not

to respond. She didn't pursue it either, snapping off her gloves and telling me my vagina and cervix looked "medically uncomplicated." I didn't know what that meant, but I took it as a sign that nothing was amiss. There was nothing to see here. We would wait for the smear results to confirm that diagnosis. She took some blood, filled out some paperwork, and sent me on my way.

Now I was back for the follow up, waiting to learn why I was feeling so outside of myself. In anticipation of this visit, I had prepared a list of symptoms that had been plaguing me of late. Included on this list:

- feelings of melancholy
- confusion
- depression
- exhaustion
- unusual food cravings (pickled beets? For real.)
- waning sex drive followed by voracious libido and unexpected desire to stab my husband in eye with a pencil because the napkin he used to wipe face rustled too loudly.

Every possible diagnosis played out on a loop in my mind in the weeks since I had gone for the blood and urine tests. Brain tumour. Diabetes. Fatty liver disease. Early onset dementia. I was 41. Old enough to know better when it comes to diet and exercise and too young to give up on life.

Finally, the doctor walked into the room, her nose buried in my file folder. She sat on a stool, flipping pages and scanning their contents. She was making small noises: hmmms, ohs, and tsks.

"How are you feeling?" she asked when she finally decided to acknowledge my presence.

"Okay, I guess. Today."

She nodded. Pursed her lips. Consulted my chart again.

"You have to lose weight."

I looked at the floor, more interested in the pattern in the utilitarian tiles than in making eye contact with my healthcare provider. I've heard this lazy diagnosis my whole life. Lose the weight and all your problems will disappear.

"But you know that already," she continued. "For now, all your test results are good. Cholesterol, glucose, and blood pressure are all in the normal range."

"That's a relief," I said.

"Yeah, okay, but only for maybe four years. Or five. Then things will change." She crossed one leg over the other and glared at me. "Only make small changes to start. If you don't, you'll be sorry."

I nodded, but said nothing.

"Now, for the other things. Your thyroid is normal. White blood cells are good, too. But your hormones levels are different."

"Different? How? What does that mean?"

"Perimenopause. Very early stages."

I opened my mouth to say something, but closed it again. I had no idea what to ask. I knew nothing about menopause or its various stages. The life-changing, years-long stretch of whacked-out hormones was the farthest thing from my mind.

"That is probably why you feel crazy."

"Aren't I, like, too young?"

"No such thing. Only a male doctor will tell you that. Nobody knows why some start early or some have periods at 62."

"I'll have to ask my mother when she started peri-menopause."

"Why? Is she a doctor?"

"No," I said. "Isn't my mother's experience an indicator of what I might experience?"

"Another male story. Every woman is different. I can give you papers that will tell you some of the things that might happen."

She handed me some photocopied pages stapled together. I glanced at the titles — *Managing Menopause*, *Let's Talk About Change,* and *Understanding Early Menopause* — without absorbing what I was seeing.

My mind bounced between thoughts like a pinball.

How long until I no longer get my period?

At least I'm not going crazy.

Maybe we should have sushi for dinner tonight.

What happens next?

Did I turn off the stove before I left the house?

The randomness of some of these thoughts was alarming and I struggled to bring myself back into the present.

"So what do I need to do?"

"There is nothing you can do," my doctor said. "Pay attention to your periods. Keep track. Remind yourself that you might not always be in control of your thoughts or moods."

"I am already very aware of that. At least I know I don't have brain cancer."

"That, we don't know."

I stared at her, mouth open, waiting for my doctor to say something that would ease my mind. She remained stoically silent, staring back at me with raised eyebrows that I interpreted as "Time's up. You need to go."

"What else do I need to I do?" I asked as I pulled on my coat.

"Tell your husband. This will be harder on him than it will be on you."

TWO

HORMONES

My husband, Jeff, didn't really get to know me until we had been married for almost 12 years. Our romance was a whirlwind. Once I had ended my very unloving first marriage, I bought a computer and signed up for an online dating platform. As a newly single woman determined not to make the same mistakes, I knew what I wanted. I read between the lines and something about Jeff's profile screamed EXTREMELY HONEST AND PATIENT (that would be handy later). The first month of our courtship was talking on the phone, often late into the night. Jeff had a hectic travel schedule, and it took a month for us to co-ordinate a night to actually meet in person for dinner. Finally, we found a date that worked, but then his flight home to Toronto from Edmonton was delayed. He offered to take the red-eye flight and keep our date. It was a lovely gesture, but I declined. It was also a clear indication of what kind of man he is.

Our actual first date took place at my favourite sushi restaurant. We sat in a private room, on cushioned tatami mats. The conversation flowed freely. From the moment I met Jeff, I felt I could be candid about everything. I didn't feel the need to present him with any fake version of myself. I was honest and open and it was refreshing. We laughed, we ate, and we planned a second date.

A month after our first date, we were pregnant. It wasn't an accident, but it wasn't exactly planned with precision. We were both in that stage of life where we knew what we wanted and could quickly identify the things that didn't work. Jeff and I fit together.

Everything about our life together was on fast forward. We moved in together, officially, three months after meeting. We were married four months after that, and our first child arrived three months after that. If you are having trouble with the timeline, we met online, got married, and had our first kid over the span of 11 months.

My pregnancy was easy and unremarkable. My fine hair grew thick and luxurious. My hips finally fulfilled their destiny, supporting my growing stomach with stability and strength. My food aversions were limited to meat; my cravings exclusively focused on ice cream. During my last trimester, Jeff gained 20 pounds, the result of daily trips to the ice cream shop. Pregnancy was a joyous time for me. I loved having company all the time, even if the communication was one way. Every flutter, kick and in utero hiccup made me smile. Unlike some women, my hormone fluctuations were unremarkable. Only once in the 39 weeks of my first pregnancy did my laughter devolve into hysterical tears. I may have occasionally been quick to anger, but I was mostly aglow with the anticipation of meeting our child. Jeff felt the same. We were partners in everything: choosing names, buying the furniture and supplies, wondering what life would be like with a baby.

When we brought Mason home from the hospital and

placed our sleeping baby in his crib, I looked at Jeff and asked, "Now what?"

He shrugged. "Are you hungry?"

I paused for moment, taking in the tiny human with the twitchy arms.

"Yeah, I actually am," I answered.

"McDonald's?"

I smiled. For the first time in almost 10 months, I wanted to sink my teeth into a greasy, salty, Quarter Pounder with cheese. Suggesting hangover food might have been his intuition, a reflection of how he was feeling, or just dumb luck. We sat in silence on the couch with our burgers, fries, and diet Cokes, both of us lost in the monumental moment of becoming parents.

We settled comfortably into parenthood. We fumbled together, figuring out what the heck we were doing. We supported each other when exhaustion set in, watching silly movies while Mason fed into the wee hours of the night. At times, I felt like a Hot Pocket in the microwave, ready to blow at any minute. A perfectly calm afternoon could spiral into me pacing in our galley kitchen in our condominium, yelling about the delay in mail delivery.

"It's a route they follow, right? It seems simple to me," I shouted, throwing my hands up in the air. "If you go to the same places every day, why do you deliver by noon one day and not until 4 p.m. the next?"

Jeff knew better than to try to reason with me or calm me down. He nodded his agreement and waited until I was finished before distracting me by nuzzling my neck and telling me how much he loved my passion. He was patient and kind when I took over with an attitude of "mother knows best" and let him know, with an air of snarky superiority, that he needed to close the diaper on the left side first. I can see now how ridiculous I had become.

I joined parenting forums online and made some friends who had babies the same age as ours. When we went offline and met in real life, we got together for large dinner parties — five couples plus the babies — and we shared all the goofiness and insecurities that come with being a first-time parent. My mommy friends and I were hormonal equals, forgiving of each other's post-natal moodiness. As we walked malls together, bought ridiculous Halloween costumes as a group, and had playdates at each other's houses, we had a safe space to be irrational when we needed to be and a sympathetic ear for venting about everything from boob milk stains to cars without car seats parked in the mommy spots.

Our last group dinner happened in January 2005, two months before Jeff's job gave us the opportunity to move from Toronto to Calgary and two weeks before we discovered I was pregnant again. I was just five months into my postpartum journey. My hair had barely had a chance to fall out before it started to shine again. My moods were still not stable. I could spiral from anger to despair in the space of four breaths. In the mid-morning, I would be excited about the new baby; by late afternoon I hated that my existing baby would not go down for a nap. I attempted to stabilize myself by going on walks with the stroller, stopping at the McDonald's 450 metres down the road for a cheeseburger fix.

For the next seven months, life was a roller coaster. We moved to a city where we knew nobody. Jeff continued to travel for work and I was home alone with one under a year and another on the way. My life went from fun-filled socializing to isolation and loneliness. Every feeling was exaggerated by pregnancy. And then, after the birth of our second son, those feelings continued to be exacerbated by post-partum hormones. But this time I was alone.

Once again, I turned to my computer for help. I found an online community of moms in Calgary and began to build friendships that would later transpire into real life. The moms doled out advice about how to manage with two under two.

"Get them on the same nap schedule."

"Deal with crises one at a time."

"Forget the housework and take a nap."

"Get out of the house."

I had to learn how to juggle two babies. I had no choice. As a social person in a hormonal flux, that isolation felt made me feel like I was dying a little every day. I figured out how to nurse a six-week-old Westin in his baby carrier while I helped Mason walk the balance beam at gymnastics.

Shortly before the end of class, while the children were playing under a parachute, one of the other moms approached me.

"Excuse me, but were you breastfeeding your baby during class?"

I gazed at this woman with the bouncy bob, wire-framed cat-eye glasses, and perfectly applied mascara.

Instinctively, I went on the defence.

"Yes," I said assertively. "He gets hungry, I feed him."

Her eyes met mine, then flicked down to Westin, who was gazing at me with his unfocused and sleepy big blue eyes.

The woman smiled so wide, I could see her molars.

"You are amazing," she exclaimed.

Without warning, I burst into tears. It was so abrupt

and forceful, a blob of snot flew out of my nose and landed on the carpet.

With the calm of someone who has seen this before, she pulled a packet of tissues out of her jeans pocket and handed me one. She took out a second one and used it to clean my snot bubble from the floor.

She stood beside me as I reined in my tears. I didn't want Mason to emerge from the polyester parachute and see his mom bawling.

"I'm Jocelyn[1]," she said. "I think we're going to be friends. Now, can I hold that baby?"

She was right. For the next three years, we became each other's lifeline. I took in her children when she had back surgery; she entertained my kids at her home while I worked to build a business. We built a bubble of safety around us, a space where we could share everything without fear of judgment. Between Jocelyn and Jeff, I had two very stable supports. Day by day, I felt my post-pregnancy hormones levelling out. Then, Jeff was offered a position we couldn't turn down, and we were on the move again, this time to Vancouver. My emotional roller coaster was back at full-tilt, but this time driven by boredom and loneliness instead of hormones. It was during our three years in Vancouver that I found the doctor who diagnosed my peri-menopause. But before that diagnosis came, while Jeff was entrenched in his new and demanding job, I was spiralling downward. Jeff had married an outgoing, energetic woman with a wicked sense of humour. I was turning into a critical, get-off-me, memory-challenged wreck.

----

1. Name has been changed because we are no longer friends and I don't want an awkward conversation.

THREE

PERIMENOPAUSE CALENDAR

Throughout university and my professional career, I kept track of my life with a luxury leather-bound daytimer. I loved making lists, tracking essay due dates and appointments, and flipping the tabs in the address book section. My choice of layout was one day per page, with a lined column on the left hand side where I could make notes. It was at the top of this column where I tracked my periods with a simple capital "P" marking Day 1. At the end of every year, I recycled the calendar portion, tossing away the record.

The digital calendar was a huge adjustment for me. I was slow to adopt one and adapt to it, but as a mom of two babies in diapers, carrying a bulky book was no longer an option. I first tried to switch to a wallet-sized paper calendar I found at the dollar store, but those found their way out of the diaper bag and into Westin's mouth, or as colouring pages for Mason, or as a butt cleaner when I forgot to replenish my supply of baby wipes. I had to make a digital calendar work for me and I'm glad I finally did.

Digitally keeping track of everything means I can look

back in time, at any time. Unlike my paper history that was tossed annually, a digital calendar allows me to confirm that, yes, my last period started January 10, 2017. The period before that was on September 28, 2016. The one before that was August 20, 2016, only 17 days after the one before that on August 3.

Prepare yourselves ladies. The red days on your calendar will no longer be periodic (sorry), but more episodic and just as predictable as a volcanic eruption. If I scroll back through my calendar, it paints a picture of how much of my life needed to be noted and sorted. But it also shows the evolution of my life from stay-at-home mom to business owner, and I am damn proud of that. I'm grateful for my digital diary, because there were things that had been completely wiped from my memory.

Thanks to my calendar, I know the menopause conversation with my doctor happened on December 13, 2010. My calendar at that time was populated with normal events: playdates, appointments, work schedule, committee meetings, and kids' activities. As I scroll through the months, I can see when things started to change. Less than six months after that "you're in perimenopause" assessment, I was noting everything in my calendar, even the minutiae: signing papers, calls to make, and bills to pay. If something wasn't noted in my calendar, there was a good chance I would completely forget about it.

As my periods became more irregular, so did the annotations and appointments in my calendar. Things like "Appraisal Larry," "Questions for Joey," and an entry to "Buy sweetener" that was not attached to any grocery list and was the only thing on my schedule that day, were noted and scheduled. The more I adjusted to using a digital calendar, the more detailed my entries became. Many of them included links to maps or websites. In the notes for my hairdresser appointments, I added photos of cut and colour options. I typed out topics of conversation for playdates and business meetings, like I couldn't trust that I would have anything of value to contribute if I didn't have notes to refer to.

My to-do lists included details such as: clean out backpacks, clean pile in kitchen, and, curious to me now, the times and dates of TV shows I wanted to watch. Clicking through the days is like opening a time capsule long forgotten. It is filled with names of people I can't even remember who must have passed into my life for a moment and then never again. There is evidence of networking events I don't recall attending, either because I didn't go or it was so mundane my brain wiped it from memory. The most intriguing curiosity is an eight-week Sunday afternoon course of taekwondo at the YMCA that I don't remember taking. My kids confirm that neither of them took that either.

If I look carefully enough at my calendar, I can also track which of my friends' marriages went sour. "Dinner with the Coultons" evolved into "Lunch with Sarah C." "Coffee with Lisa Megg" in April became "Coffee with Lisa (Megg) Jacobs" in October. At the time, I hadn't noticed just how many of my baby-days friends' marriages were no longer intact. I do recall a lot of "trial separations," but we moved before I could follow those storylines to the finish. It's hard to watch your friends spiral into the ugly bits of divorce. I was lucky. My own divorce from my first husband happened way before I was even close to my hormonal breakdown and was simple and quick.

My perimenopause lasted for six years, from the age of 41 until my last period before I turned 47. Over the course of that time, we moved from British Columbia, returning to Ontario and then made our way back to Alberta. The transitions didn't exaggerate my symptoms, but they kept me distracted while we unpacked boxes and got familiar with a new neighbourhood. When we moved back to Toronto, I was unsettled and emotional, partly from constantly being in interprovincial movement, partly from the first year in perimenopause, and partly from struggling with our youngest son's diagnosis of attention deficit disorder. I had placed so much hope on the move back to Toronto. Having grown up and spent a good portion of my adult life there, I was looking forward to being back in the city I knew. I had envisioned our kids getting to know their grandparents. I was looking forward to social gatherings again. But the real estate market had changed since we moved from Toronto to Vancouver and on our return, the only home we could afford was 45 minutes north of the city limits and an hour and a half one-way commute to work for Jeff. We were so far removed from the life I imagined.

While I can't remember my exact thoughts, I can still feel how untethered I was from everyone and everything. I felt alone and resentful and I took it out on everyone when I wasn't shoving junk food in my mouth. My middle was filling out, not just from menopausal settling, but from trying to drown my feelings under a Quarter Pounder with cheese. I put on my happy mask, but inside I was boiling over.

When we moved back to Calgary a little more than a year later, I felt more at ease and ready to go back to the city that felt more like home than Toronto did. I was finding my way back to my business and my friends and enjoying the strong bond we had as a family. Even in the throes of periods that were all over the map, emotional instability, and unrelenting memory issues, I got better at holding on to the things that brought me joy. With age and menopause comes an awareness of who you are, what's important, and who matters in your life. So be assured, while you cannot control anything that is happening hormonally, you can be confident that you will get through this, emerging stronger and wiser (and wider) on the other side.

FOUR

MOOD MADNESS

The first inkling that something was really wrong happened when I looked at my husband sitting on the couch watching TV and I had a random thought.

I could murder you right now for no reason other than you are in the same room as me.

Rage pushed against my chest, trying to burst out like an alien baby. I clenched my teeth, balled my hands into fists, and tried not to look at him. The muscles in my face involuntarily worked themselves into a scowl of disgust. In my heart, I knew this was unfounded, but in my head I felt that if I had quick access to a knife, I would have stabbed my husband.

I kept my lips tightly sealed in a grimace. I didn't move. I let the bitterness and resentment work its way through my body. I didn't know why this was happening, but I knew it wasn't me. This was something else entirely.

Mood swings during perimenopause are exactly what you think they would be. Irrational. Flashing by like a strobe light. Unexpected, uncontrollable, and unwarranted. The last time my emotions controlled me with such volatility was when I was 15 years old and rebellious as heck, just like everyone else I hung out with. My pregnancy hormones paled in comparison to these wild fluctuations. This time, I had no one around me who felt the same way, or even talked about feeling off kilter.

Even before that killer instinct hit me in the living room, I would tear up over commercials about cars and ice cream. Taylor Swift's song *Never Grow Up* would reduce me to a puddle of tears. I would rant over the injustice of Netflix US getting better content than Netflix Canada. I felt overwhelmed by the simple act of emptying the dishwasher. That feeling could be followed by absolute triumph when I weeded the garden.

For the better part of three years, I was mostly angry and it was entirely the fault of my waning estrogen and progesterone. I mostly kept it to myself, recognizing that it was unfair to unleash my wrath on my husband and children. Sometimes, however, I would lose control and lose my mind over the smallest of infractions, not all of which were deliberate actions. Spilled juice would descend into a bluster about carelessness, waste, and the inequitable division of household duties. Tech that didn't work as it should turned me into a raving idiot threatening to move the whole family to an off-grid cabin in the woods. Socks that got stuck to the inside of sweatpants set me off on a misguided mission to turn all pants inside out looking for errant socks.

My mood wasn't just restricted to the basics of anger or sadness. There was another symptom, an unexpected by-product of hormone changes and brain chemistry fluctuations. It crept up on me. For the first time in my life, I was plagued with feelings of anxiety about how long I had left to live. I thought about my death, obsessing over the fact that I was very likely at the halfway point of my life. Day or night, I worried about mortality, and not just my own. I chewed my nails when my husband added butter to his mashed potatoes, silently building a survival scenario should he die before me. When my children went out, I had visions of them being run over and mangled by a truck while riding their bikes to school. I found myself imagining a car launching over the highway median and crushing me. The images in my head were so vivid, my heart would start racing and I would sweat. I would lose focus for a whole day, waiting for my kids and husband to return home safe. I had to stop watching disaster movies because the worst scenarios would work themselves into my psyche. I pictured earthquakes opening a hole to the netherworld in my kitchen. I envisioned my children innocently sitting in the school cafeteria, laughing with their friends until the roof was ripped off the building and a Sharknado pulled them all to a bloody, toothy death.

All this was happening in privacy. I didn't talk to anyone. I didn't share my anxiety. I ate my feelings — the crunchier the crutch, the better. I avoided nuts and other choking hazards because those could trigger more imagined death scenarios. As I got to the bottom of another bag of chips, I made a mental note to seek professional help or ask my doctor about what I was feeling. Like many women, however, I pushed my concerns aside and put my own health on the back burner.

A 43-year-old friend of mine, Christine, also had visions of horrible things happening to her family.

"I thought I was going crazy," she told me. "When I would tell my husband about my fears of something bad happening to the kids, he would tell me that I needed to loosen up and that my mind was playing tricks on me."

This is not helpful advice for a woman experiencing perimenopause and will likely result in circling right back to the kind of murderous thoughts from the beginning of this chapter.

When my friend Valery was diagnosed with peri-menopause at the age of 44, her doctor recommended an IUD (intra-uterine device) to stem the severe bleeding and cramping brought on by hormonal changes.

"After five years my doctor removed the IUD and then full menopause hit," Valery said. "All at once I had all the symptoms. Hot flashes every hour, not sleeping, and I was a bitch every second of every day. The mood swings were dramatic and I wasn't a very nice person to be around, but only to my husband. Nobody else noticed how I had become, or if they did, they didn't say anything."

Yvonne experienced a significant flip in her personality when she had a full hysterectomy at age 43, due to a uterine prolapse.

"I got menopause on a plate in one serving. My before and after was very, very clear," she said. In the space of one day, Yvonne went from being an active, healthy, and vibrant wife, mother, and business owner to a sad, depressed, and lonely woman.

"My bones hurt, my joints hurt, my hair fell out, my nails all broke. My skin was sallow, I could not move well, could not walk well. I sat in a chair, staring out the window. I wasn't crying, just hopeless."

On any given day, my pendulous moods swung wildly from happiness to rage, then from rage to melancholy, from melancholy to romantic. Managing my mood swings during perimenopause was like alternately dealing with a petulant child and a raving lunatic. Somehow, in the middle of my temporary insanity, the voice of reason was able to break through. Almost three years into perimenopause, I had a moment when I came as close to an out-of-body experience as I ever have. Sitting on the couch, simmering with discontent, I felt my logical mind pull away from the cloud of irrationality. That clarity allowed the voice to whisper: *This isn't a real feeling. This is your eggs dying off. This is The Change.*

Phew. So I wasn't a murderous bitch after all.

FIVE

PERIODS

Warning: If the image of the uterus above didn't already indicate there might be some graphic material, I'll spell it out. In the spirit of being honest and candid, I need to share some really gross things. If you don't like blood — hearing about it, reading about it, or envisioning it — then proceed with caution into this chapter. I'm not capable of using euphemisms for body parts or menstruation. I left that to my mother, who insisted her vibrator was a massager.

༁

I was blessed with mostly predictable and uncomplicated periods. I started when I was 12, which was a relief, given that I knew my mother started when she was 10 years old. I had a normal and uneventful development, from training bra to real bra, and from pads to tampons.

For the whole of my adult life, my periods came every 25 or 26 days, with few exceptions. I paid attention to my period calendar and even if I didn't, my PMS symptoms would let me know it was almost time. I know I was blessed to be so regular. Until perimenopause, my period was just something to deal with and plan around on a monthly basis. But no matter my cycle, I clearly remember three critical period events:

1. That one time I lost track and my period showed up unexpectedly when at a party, on a date, or about to have sex.
2. That one time I had unprotected sex, or the condom broke, or he swore he pulled out in time and my period was late for the first time ever.
3. That one time my period was late when I wanted it to be and was on the high of realizing I was making a baby.

From the onset of my period, my cramps were manageable with Midol or Tylenol or Advil. Day 1 brought the worst cramps, but as long as I was medicated, I could manage to carry on with my life. I watched my mother struggle her whole life with crippling menstrual cramps and I was so grateful for not having to suffer like that. My flow was a little heavier on Day 2, but nothing like some of my peers who had to back up their tampon with pads to staunch the flow. These were things I didn't discover until I was an adult, because back in the 1980s and 1990s, nobody openly talked about their periods. The most vocal anyone got was at summer camp when a newbie would shout out, "Anyone have a pad or a tampon?" from the washhouse.

I hated pads from the outset. They were bulky, and the feeling of perpetual wetness in my underpants grossed me out. Pads did nothing to mask the musky menstrual odour and the scented ones made me feel like I was a walking air freshener that had gone slightly off. Before there were wings, leaks were common and mortifying for a teenager. One summer afternoon, I discovered just how absorbent my pads were when I decided to go swimming with one stuck to the gusset of my Speedo. I dived into the deep end of the pool and before I could break the surface I felt the weighted mass of my pad pulling my swimsuit down. I swam to the shallow end, trying to determine if I could get out of the pool without anyone noticing the sag and bulk between my legs. I then half swam, half dog-paddled back to the deep end to get closer to where my towel lay and used the ladder to climb out. Within seconds, I had my towel wrapped around my waist and, with pink-tinged water pouring down my legs, made it to the change room without having to suffer the humiliation of a fellow teen noticing and asking if I was wearing a diaper. That was an experiment that was never going to be repeated.

I endured the cramps and the cravings. I learned to ignore the stupid boys who would jeer, "Are you on the rag?" when I wore my period sweatpants or was just in a pissy mood. I shook my head in horror when my mom asked me if I needed her to show me how to use a tampon. As an adult building my career, I spent more than one lunch hour racing to the drugstore for supplies.

I can't pinpoint when I realized my standard-issue ovaries started running the show like toddlers in a ball pit — reckless, with crazed abandon and the unexpected release of bodily fluids. But for three years before I was fully menopausal, my period started to go wacky. The 26-day cycle became more of a roulette wheel than a reliable calendar. As I moved further into perimenopause, there was nothing regular about my periods.

My periods began to come 32 days apart, or 21 days

apart, or whenever the heck they felt like coming. The shortest span was 15 days from the start of one to the start of the next and the longest window was 49 days. There were days when I felt the telltale signs of my period — gentle cramping, sore boobs, a need to feed — but nothing more would happen. One evening, I jumped up from the dinner table after my uterus contracted and I felt a warm wetness between my legs. In the bathroom, a clotted smear of blood lined my underpants. I cleaned myself up and grabbed a tampon. When I went to change the tampon a few hours later, there was a single brown spot on one side of the tampon, barely the size of a pea. I stared at the spot, the tampon dangling in front of me like a cotton pendulum, wondering what the hell was happening to my body. As I sat on the toilet, my mind went sideways. *Should I go to the doctor? Do I have cancer? Do I put another tampon in?*

I decided to wear a tampon that night. In the morning, the thing was still dry. Not a drop of blood. Erratic periods wasn't something my friends and I discussed openly. When I asked my mother, she replied that I was too young for menopause and that she didn't remember anything about hers anyways.

Other women who have been completely regular with their cycles, have found perimenopause wreaked the worse kind of havoc with their flow. Carrie, age 50, went from regular flow to "slaughter-like periods." Sandra[1], at age 52, went 61 days without a period and woke up on Day 62 in a blood-soaked bed.

"I had been a regular, every 28-day kind of girl since the age of 12," she wrote.

----

2. Name changed upon request. I don't blame her. That's a very disturbing event that belongs in a Stephen King novel.

"I took my first (and hopefully) last pregnancy test at the age of 51. Then my period came like a blood bath.

Thank god for mattress protectors because I woke up in a literal pool."

For me, the cycle numbers were so random, I took the last six cycles and played the numbers in the lottery.

15, 21, 26, 33, 36, 49.

I won a free play and $2.

SIX

PHYSICAL UNFITNESS

In my second year of perimenopause, we bought an elliptical machine. It wasn't an impulse buy. Over the course of our marriage, my husband and I have taken turns deciding what fitness equipment we would purchase. Just after we had our second child, I chose a treadmill. For a while, I diligently went down to the basement at 5 a.m., baby monitor in hand, to use it. After three weeks, my adorable little babies decided 6 a.m. was a sleep-in and started rousing themselves around 5:15 a.m. I'm sure they had internal sensors that let them know Mommy wasn't on the same floor and it was time to cry. For the next two years, the treadmill sat abandoned until we moved to British Columbia. In our new home, I used the treadmill to start running. This was another short-term program, not because our kids interrupted me, but because I discovered I hated running.

My husband chose the elliptical machine. The day the elliptical was installed in our upstairs media/fitness room, Jeff was out of town. It was my duty to decide where in the room the machine would be positioned. My only requirement was that it be situated in such a way so I could watch television and hopefully forget I wasn't having a good time.

I stood in front of the machine, hands clenched into fists, staring at my nemesis. I pursed my lips and tilted my head, studying the machine for any sign of weakness. No matter what it took, I was going to make this machine my bitch.

I started with short workouts, gradually increasing the length of time and intensity. I had to throw a towel over the display so I didn't have to look at the hateful information confirming I'd been in motion for only six minutes, not 45 as anticipated. I had some very satisfying workouts for eight months and then the dust started building up. After three years of living in solitude in the spare bedroom, the elliptical was given away and Jeff and I agreed to invest in a recumbent bike. With its shiny handles and interactive display, the bike had no inkling it would suffer the same fate as its predecessors.

Physical fitness has never been my strong suit. Every piece of equipment that has come into my home was greeted with enthusiasm. *This* was going to be the thing that worked. I was ready for the challenge and looked forward to overcoming the obstacles my mind put in the way. I was attracted to the lights, the shiny chrome, and the Bluetooth connectivity. I committed quickly, but the glow of a healthy relationship dimmed, morphing into hurling mental insults at myself, even though I agreed to the purchase and was 100 per cent involved in its selection. Maybe things would have worked out better if a sushi dinner were involved.

There are a couple of common threads weaving through every fitness purchase:

1. My husband never stepped foot on anything we bought.
2. Despite my best efforts and dedicated schedule, I never lost a single pound.

I'd just about given in, resigned to be unfit forever. But I don't give up that easily. In the midst of trying to figure out what was happening to my body, I had a wonderful business lunch at a vegan restaurant. The conversation was great and the food was delicious. I felt the fog lift from my brain and I was on a creative high. Instead of acknowledging that I was hungry and the food was the nourishment I needed, I took this as a sign that becoming vegetarian was going to be my fix. I swore off meat for the next six months, until a plate of saucy and spicy chicken wings beckoned me back. I cried a bit after the first bite. It felt like a reunion of sorts, like picking your child up from their first sleepover or retrieving your pet post-vacation from the kennel: you were glad for the break, but man, did you miss them. My brief stint as a non-carnivore let my brain live somewhere else for a while but had no effect on my body shape, weight, or mental state.

SEVEN

BODY CHANGES

Much like pregnancy, perimenopause steals control of your body. Things grow where they shouldn't, parts give up the fight against gravity, and sections expand without any external encouragement.

The most sensible way to outline exactly what happened to me is to start at the top.

HAIR HERE, THERE, AND EVERYWHERE

I've always had extremely fine hair. During my early tween years, I allowed my mother to convince me a perm was the way to go. It would give my hair some body, she said. It will be easy to take care of, she explained. Simply wash and go. While that was true, I wanted to fan and flip my hair like the other girls. I wanted a ponytail or some braids. I didn't want my hair to always look like it belonged to beardless Bob Ross.

My hair had always been stringy and mousy and as soon

as I had money in my pocket, I made a big change. At the age of 15, I swore off perms, dyed my hair bright orange, and had it cut so I could slick it back or gel and spray it up in spikes. It wasn't until my first pregnancy that I experienced the kind of hair I had always dreamed about. By the end of my first trimester, my hair was thick and lush and stayed that way until postpartum hormones kicked in and my hair started to return to its former self. I nipped that in the bud by getting pregnant again.

As perimenopause crept into my life, I noticed my hair was thinning out even more, except for the grey. The grey hairs that were sprouting from the centre of my scalp and at my temples were thick and curly. No matter how much product I used, there was almost always a cluster of wiry, kinky greys sticking to the side of my temple like a steel wool scrubber. While I once could go a few days without washing my hair, my overactive hormones made my hair greasy and limp in less than a day. I noticed my hairline was receding and a small bald spot was forming on the back of my head.

My hair not only was falling out, it was migrating. Once, while pulling my hair back into a ponytail, I felt a sharp tug on my ear lobe. I'd caught my new ear hair as I swept my hair back. It was that long. I was horrified. Would I now have to buy a hair trimmer for my nose and ears? Did they even come in pink?

As I progressed further toward menopause, I noticed I was looking more like my father: less hair on top, more hair on my face. Plucking my chin hairs has become a regular part of grooming. I am almost obsessed with getting these bastards out. While I'm in my car where the light is good, I'll sit at a stoplight or in the driveway plucking the hairs and pinching out the blackheads. A friend of mine once posted a snarky update on Facebook, calling out the "disgusting" woman in the car beside her who was plucking away. *It could have been me,* I thought. I was about to respond to her post with "It will happen to you too, missy," but I didn't want to rob her of the delightful realization that one day she too will need to do something about her menopause beard.

Periodically, a chin hair plays an elusive game of hide and seek with me. I can feel it with my fingertips, but it hasn't emerged enough for me to grasp it with tweezers. I'll tug on it with my fingernails, but it slips away. When I finally do get it, the satisfaction is so deep I take a moment to look at the hair, like a victor assessing the spoils of war.

I've begun investing in facial wax strips. My face has a downy dusting of hair now. It's light and barely noticeable, except on the sides of my face where the hair is darker and, if not tended to, might lead to mutton chops. This new fur has clearly come from my legs and armpits, which no longer require weekly shaves. I have to change the blade on my razor not from use, but from the rust that builds as it sits abandoned on the shower shelf.

ABOUT FACE

It is a cruel joke to look in the mirror in my mid-to-late forties and see every season of life staring back at me. On any given day, my menopausal hormones will work together to make my wrinkles look deeper while simultaneously producing the largest zit I've had in 25 to 30 years. It's a confusing self-portrait: grey hair at the temples, laugh lines radiating out from the eyes, and a red, angry pimple erupting from the middle of your hairy chin.

All this aging glory comes with some additional features: sagging and filling. My eyelids started to droop and get crepey, providing a channel for my makeup to migrate from my lids and lashes into the bags under my eyes. No wonder people always said I look tired. The skin on the lower half of my face started to sag while my jowls started to look fuller.

An age spot appeared on my right cheek. It stands out like the superstorm on Jupiter because it's set against the backdrop of dull skin and crater-sized pores. I have always been a makeup minimalist, having watched my mother apply heavy, almost comical makeup her whole life, but during perimenopause I became keenly interested in foundation. With the change in my skin tone, I had the perfect excuse to find some new lipsticks and try as many foundation samples as was allowed.

In my last year of perimenopause, I headed to Sephora under the assumption that the selection would be much better than the drugstore. Plus, Sephora staff will basically hold your hand if you want them to and this was not an adventure I felt equipped to manage without any help. The last time I had bought an entire new line of makeup was when I was 22. I had my father's credit card and his blessing to buy whatever I wanted for my birthday. I spent over an hour at the Chanel counter in Saks Fifth Avenue and walked away with everything from foundation (which my cousin exclaimed made my skin look "like a porcelain doll!") to lipstick. I even added an eyeshadow brush and a blush brush, both of which I still have. My dad's shock still rings in my ears: "You spent $400 on makeup?" Yeah, I did. It was my Julia Roberts in *Pretty Woman* moment.

This time around, it was my own coin and I was far less interested in glam and more concerned about blending my aging away. Delicately. I wasn't going to be one of those women who cakes on the makeup every day until the funeral director takes over. Sephora makes me happy and I'm not sure why. Maybe it's the lighting. I know the lights are deliberately flattering and evenly spaced throughout the store. The fixtures are lit and the whole place is meant to mirror lighting variations in real life. Before Sephora, we all bought makeup at department store counters where the fluorescents made everyone look bad, but made it easier to see how makeup could transform your face. Maybe the magic of Sephora was in the clusters of women trying lipsticks and "oohing" and "ahhing" with their friends. Or it could be the cheery young ladies walking the sales floor swinging baskets over their arms like they are ready to take you on a makeover picnic (they are).

I walked into the makeup superstore filled with hope. I couldn't stop staring at the associate who spoke to me first. I'm not sure what she said because I was so distracted by the painted perfection on her face. She likely spends more time applying her makeup than I do searching my chin for rogue hairs.

"Ma'am, are you okay?"

I snapped out of my reverie. I opened my mouth to protest the ageism in calling me ma'am, then promptly shut it again so I could smile. In this place, I *was* a ma'am by about 20 years.

"I'm good, thanks," I said.

"Can I help you find anything?"

I started to shake my head and took a few steps away, but then I stopped. *If I'm direct with my needs, this can be a quick trip.*

"I'm looking for foundation," I started and then listed

my orders like a drill sergeant. "I don't want anything too heavy. No powder. I don't want to feel it on my face. It can't smell. I need it to hide my pores not clog them. It has to be easy to apply. One step."

I took a step back to get a good look at her face. I knew she was searching the waters of the makeup database in her mind, splashing around in the deep end of the pool. Just when I thought all was lost, her glossy lips broke into a smile.

"I think I know what you need. Right this way."

I suspected she was going to escort me to the door, pat me on the back, and wish me the best of luck. Instead, she put her basket away, brought her hands together under her chin like she was praying, and studied my face.

"Let's go to a mirror," she announced as she clapped her hands, like this was the best idea she'd had *evah*.

We crossed from the outside lanes of the store into the middle. She examined my face in the light and it didn't feel uncomfortable. I liked the attention. I felt like this might be fun.

I'd been out of the makeup loop so long that there were now more brands than I could count. She was so focused on solving my problem that I felt like handing over my credit card and telling her to get me whatever I needed. I couldn't understand why I had this absolute trust in a complete stranger.

One by one, foundation swatches were applied in gentle circular motions. After the first 10 minutes, my face was spotted with so many different samples, I looked like a hyena with mange. Over the next 45 minutes, we tried all the wrong things. I couldn't land on anything that solved my problem and ticked all my comfort boxes. I admired the young lady for her tenacity and I wondered if she felt like she was playing with her Barbie doll. For a fleeting second, my menopausal mind veered off-course, wondering if Mattel would make a middle-aged Barbie. If they filled out the hips, brought the boobs down, and added a wine stain to her maxi dress, she'd be the most real she's ever been.

Finally, I put my hand up and asked her to stop. I assessed the carnage of foundation bottles and compacts, tissues, blotting papers, cotton pads, and disposable applicators. I wiped my face clean of any remaining product. I turned to my fearless foundation brush wielder and asked, "Where is the NARS?"

We walked one aisle back to the NARS display. She bent down to look at the selection. She pulled out two sample bottles, squirted the liquid onto Q-Tips and rubbed each shade in a circle onto the fleshy part of my hand between my thumb and forefinger.

"That's the one," I said, pointing to the sample closest to my thumb.

It really was that simple. I knew all along that I preferred NARS for my face foundation, but my brain either buried that knowledge or my judgment was clouded by all the attention I was getting.

"Is there anything else I can help you find?" Below the perfectly shaped eyebrows that may or may not have been tattooed, I could see the hope in her eyes that my answer was no. She was bored with this Barbie and didn't want to play anymore.

I paused, wondering if I wanted to subject her to more torture while I worked my way through the lipstick brands. Not too much pigment. Not sticky. Shine, but not gloss. Nude, but with colour. Winter colours and summer colours.

"Just point me to Charlotte Tilbury," I answered. "I need a lipstick."

THE SKIN I'M IN

I can't be the only who misses the skin of their youth. Once upon a time, I had a flawless complexion. I tanned evenly in the summer and when I burned, my skin turned golden brown a day later. If I cut myself, it healed within two days. Bruises were the signs of a life well-lived: hip smashing into strangers in a packed night club, stumbling into a booth at a greasy diner for a hangover breakfast, round-kicking a 300-pound boxing bag at the gym.

Menopause stole all these miracles of my skin from me. If I spend too long in the sun, I usually end up with a rash, even with ample sunscreen applied. My years of sun-worshipping with baby oil have left me with a legacy of age spots on my arms and paranoia about the skin tags on my back. We knew nothing about skin cancer and even if we did, I probably would have yielded to the ignorance of my youth in favour of spectacularly sun-kissed skin and an adorable bit of sunburn on my nose.

The skin thins out during menopause. I can look at my arms and legs and map the path of my veins from my finger-tips to my chest with only minor detours along the stretch marks. But I do need to spend money on moisturizer because my skin is so much drier than it ever was. Even when I get out of a steamy shower, the skin on my face feels like it's being pulled back behind my ears. For a few minutes, I can pretend I've had a face lift. But once the mirror clears, I can see I look less like a younger version of myself and more like Voldemort in a bathrobe. My hands and elbows crack in the winter and the patterning on my unmoisturized arms closely resembles a lizard.

Bruising these days is a result of sitting down on the couch, or lying on my side for too long, or rubbing my forearm against the mayonnaise in the fridge while I'm reaching for the pickles. The bruises are *spectacular* works of art. This one, on the outer flesh of my left knee, looks like a melted clock painted by Salvador Dali. The one on my right hand makes me think of Monet and his blobbish, blooming *Water Lilies*. The one on my abdomen has been there for so long, its swirls of blue and black and yellow now remind me of my favourite painting, van Gogh's *Starry Night*.

Our menopausal skin cannot keep up with the daily assaults of life. Rashes will manifest in skin folds, easily brought on by sweat or by the spoonful of potato salad you snuck into your mouth when you woke up just past midnight and desperately needed to eat. If you are squeamish, skip this next anecdote from Carrie, age 50.

"I had a horrid experience where I was getting my bikini line waxed," she told me. "I have had this done several times over the years. The last time I went, half my skin came up with the tape, leaving not only a long sore down my groin, but my esthetician was horrified."

Here is my sage advice: Invest in a good moisturizer, stay out of the sun, and let things grow wild from now on.

BODY MOVES

I had an hourglass figure for about three weeks when I was in my late twenties. Other than that blessed period, I have always been pear-shaped: C-cup, tapered waist, ample bottom. I was comfortable with my shape and after a candid conversation back then with a dear friend with a similar shape (except her breasts were way bigger), I stopped trying to reshape my body. I changed my wardrobe instead. I was well into my twenties when I figured out that an empire waist and A-line skirt were the best styles for my body.

"We are never going to have flat asses," she sighed as we sat on the outdoor patio of our favourite coffee shop.

I peered over the top of my steaming non-fat, no-whip, half-caff latte, took a sip and waited.

"This is the best it's ever going to get," she said. "We are in our prime. We can't spot-reduce our bodies into a different shape. We have to work with what we have. Work on getting stronger."

I've known this woman since we were 12. We've been through the very worst awkward stages life throws at us. She likes to pontificate at length. Sometimes 10 minutes will go by and she won't even realize I haven't said a word. I know her well enough to let her think out loud.

"I've done everything I can. Gym, diets, pills... I've even talked to a shrink for fuck's sake," she said.

"Yeah? How'd that go?"

"Apparently my food and eating issues are related to my dad dying when I was very young. Oh, and watching my single mom struggle to make ends meet. She said I subconsciously stuff myself because I have a fear of never having enough."

"Is that true?" I asked.

"Not at all. I am fully aware of when I'm stuffing my face."

I fucking love this woman.

"I think you're right about body shape. I always look the same, just smaller. Sometimes larger." I grinned.

"I know I'm right," she nodded.

I got up from my seat, then tossed my unfinished latte into the trash.

"Where are you going?" she asked.

"Getting a Frappuccino with loads of whipped cream. No sense fighting what I can't control."

If only I knew in my mid-twenties how sage those words were.

As I slid into menopause, everything about my body slid with it. As things sagged, the line between my waist and breasts began to blur. I know this not only because I could see it happening, but also my husband once reached over in bed and started massaging the fat roll to the left of my belly button. He seemed happy, so I didn't inform him of his error.

Like a snowbird heading for Florida in the winter, everything moves south. The abs I had before I had kids have fallen down to my hips. My knees have thickened down to my ankles. My fingernails, once strong and keratin-rich are now splitting and brittle, but my toenails can chop wood. My breasts are not only sagging down, but to the side as well. In a misguided attempt to fight gravity, I bought a push-up bra. I poured my fleshy breasts into this thing, lifting and manoeuvring them to sit nicely in the cups. Instead of giving me a subtle lift, the bra made me look like I had stuffed a ham under my shirt. To add to my horror, I glanced in the mirror as I was bent over the sink brushing my teeth and discovered I have the chest wrinkles of a bronzed grandma who spent too much time on a lounge chair in Miami.

My friend was wrong though. Our shape does change. As my middle filled out, I went from being a pear to a lumpy apple. My ass is still ample, but now everything seems oddly proportional. I have relinquished control. I no longer worry about changing my figure, but focus on building muscle. I lift weights so hefting the four-litre jug of milk onto the top shelf of the fridge doesn't cause a fainting spell. I do wall sits and squats to make going up the stairs in my home a little easier. And I do Kegels, usually while I'm sitting in the drive-thru, waiting for my half-caff-so-I-can-sleep-tonight, low-fat-to-avoid-lactose-gas Frappuccino.

EIGHT

THE AGE GAP

I woke up this morning foolishly thinking it would be a
normal day. I envisioned getting my writing done,
going to work, and having a lovely dinner with my
family. I headed to one of my favourite coffee shops, a place
where I periodically escaped to for a change of scenery from
my home office. Coffee shops, coincidentally, are wonderful
places for writers to observe and eavesdrop. My trick is to
wear my earbuds, but with nothing playing, so you think I
am not listening to you and your colleague outline the script
for the porn movie you are developing. I kid you not. I have
heard all manner of conversations in busy Starbucks cafés.
If you've ever been in a coffee shop and felt like you were
being watched, I can say with confidence it was a writer
watching how your mouth moved, how you leaned in for
emphasis and how you knocked your low-fat java chip Frappuccino over as your wildly gesturing hands became part of
the conversation. The writer also noted the moment of
panic that passed over your face as you reached out to grab
the falling cup and missed. Also registered: the relief that
washed over your flushed cheeks when you realized the cup

was already empty and you wouldn't be paying for dry cleaning the cashmere coat draped over the chair at the table right beside yours.

This is how we writers do.

And the older I get, the more I am able to blend into the background and take note.

It was on this day — this day that started like most others — that I noticed something else in my peri-menopausal world had changed. As I looked around the full coffee shop, I realized I no longer had the ability to determine anyone's age outside of my own demographic. I could pick out the tired, puffy, uncomfortable-in-this-new-stage-of-life over-40 crowd, but anyone under that age melted into an amorphous group. I was having trouble determining if the man reading *Beartown* was mid-thirties or late twenties. The young lady with the topknot and the backpack could be in her first year of university or getting ready to defend her Ph.D. Sometime in the last five years I crossed into the old people zone where everyone looks very, very, very young and I referred to anyone under 35 as "kids." Without my glasses, everyone looks like a 17-year-old.

When I was 13, I overheard my after-school babysitter inviting my mother to her 40th birthday party. I remember thinking 40 was so old and I vowed to myself I would always stay fun and vibrant. Now here I am, over 50 and wondering if 8:30 p.m. is too early to go to bed. I am standing in the middle of the middle-aged arena, surrounded by 20-somethings who think they have the answers to all of the world's problems. They are looking at me and thinking they will always make time to cover the grey hair. I can look at a young woman in her early thirties and admire her perfect makeup with the knowledge that in less than 20 years, she'll be tossing all her shimmer eye shadows and start the hunt for the perfect matte. I also know that no matter how hard you fight or how many days per week you go to the gym, sometime in your forties, your hormones will win. Your middle will pooch, your boobs will sag, and you will be sorely uncomfortable in your favourite heels. You'll wear a jacket when it's cold and don a scarf, mittens, and hat despite the good hair day because it's cold enough outside to freeze your newly grown nose hair.

I pine for the days when I thought I could rule the world. I was ambitious, full of hope, and didn't let anything get in my way. These days, when something goes awry, I am more likely to shrug my shoulders, give in, then go buy myself an ice cream. You can't win every battle, but you can always drown your sorrows in a hot fudge sundae.

NINE

WHAT DID I JUST PUT IN MY MOUTH?

I felt like I was going to puke. My stomach clenched and my bowels prepared themselves. My mouth filled with excess saliva, a sure sign that I needed to find a toilet bowl to lean over. I pressed my lips together and took deep breaths through my nose. I closed my eyes and said a silent prayer.

"Mom, are you okay?" I opened my eyes and looked at my youngest, who was sitting across from me at the dining room table. Concern washed over his face.

I nodded, afraid to speak.

A few more deep breaths and the compulsion to toss up all my dinner passed.

I took a sip of water and waited a moment to see if my stomach would object. I was fine.

"What the hell did I just eat?" I asked, gazing across the table at my husband.

He looked at his own plate, then mine, then the serving dishes in the middle of the table.

"I don't know," he said, shrugging.

On my plate were the following items: a roasted chicken breast, a dozen green beans, and some crispy roasted potatoes. Nothing offensive at all.

After questioning my husband about his choice of ingredients and spices, the realization of what made me sick became clear. It wasn't *what* I ate, it was the *taste* of what I ate. The offender: smoked paprika. For the first time in my life, a spice triggered an intolerance. This was different than the pepper chicken my husband enthusiastically over-seasoned in 2005. That time, his copious use of pepper caused a 38-week pregnant me to sneeze, breaking my water. Our second child was born 14 hours later.

Menopause can wreak havoc with your taste buds. Foods you've loved your whole life now taste different. The all-dressed chips that had been my go-to since they appeared on the market now leave a waxy film in my mouth. The tomatoes and balsamic vinegar I started eating when I lived in Italy now taste bitter and acidic.

It goes the other way too. I find myself craving pickles at any given time. I am not afraid to try strange concoctions like a cracker topped with Camembert, red pepper jelly, and an olive. Once upon a time, I would have rather licked sand than put beets in my mouth, but here I am, gobbling up a dish of pickled sweet beets as my afternoon snack.

The list of foods I could not tolerate grew longer every month. The first indulgence I had to give up was wine, particularly my beloved reds. Then it was generally any kind of alcohol. Onions, with which I have never had a close relationship, would make me burp incessantly, repeating on me over and over like any annoying song on replay. I got food poisoning from a bad banana and that horrific night left me with an intolerance to high-potassium foods such as kiwis (which I never liked anyways) and avocados (which I *loved* as long as they were found under layers of cheese, salsa, and sour cream). Red meat came off the menu after an attack of diverticulitis inflamed my intestines.

The positive side of this radical change in taste buds and tolerance is that choosing what to eat from a restaurant menu is easy. I can go two ways: I can make a choice based on what is offered or I can be a complete pain in the ass and make endless modifications to my meal. The former route is much easier and less frustrating, not just to the server, but to me as well. I have to leave my menu open because my memory is so foggy I can't remember what I wanted to order between making my initial selection and the server coming to the table to take said order. I have no desire to exacerbate that problem by

a) attempting on-demand recall of the entire list of foods I cannot eat and

b) trying to remember the eliminations from the dish I want to order.

I invariably end up ordering what caught my eye at first, taking a gamble with the fallout. My husband will be deep in sleep long before the farting starts.

The cravings I experienced would come and hold on with more tenacity than a four-year-old asking "But why?" I would wake up at 5 a.m. with my mouth watering over the idea of chicken wings. Dry-rubbed, saucy, sticky — it didn't matter. Until I could get to the pub, everything I put in my mouth that wasn't chicken wings tasted like garbage. My husband would make chicken marsala from scratch, he'd flambé fish and plate up pasta carbonara, all wonderful dishes he has mastered. Pre-cravings, I would always have seconds. I love his cooking. But with my taste buds and my brain hyper-focused on the crispy, salty, tangy chicken parts, every single dish fell flat for me. The knowledge that I couldn't even enjoy a cider with those chicken wings did not avert my focus. When the cravings hit, whether you are perimenopausal or on the other side of that hell, you have no control. The most frustrating part is the craving isn't picky about quality. If you cannot get to the pub — say your friends are all busy, your husband doesn't really want to go, or there's a pandemic forcing the closure of all restaurants — you will settle for grocery store pre-heated two-day-old chicken wings. It's a bonus if you happen to be in Toronto, a few blocks away from a grocery store that does a brisk wing business and the offerings are always fresh and tasty. My mouth is watering right now thinking about the smokin' stampede flavour with its perfect combination of barbecue sauce, spice, and vinegar. It's an absolute jackpot if the wings just came out of the fryer and there is enough to fill the family pack with four *different* flavours.

And then one day, you'll wake up, having glutted your-self on chicken wings or pasta with fake Parmesan cheese or apple slices topped with cheddar and you'll only want to eat salad. I desperately craved crispy greens. My body suddenly took great pleasure from all things vegetable. I added things to salad that I never have before, including particularly polarizing items such as raisins and beets (again with the beets!). I fell in love with kale again and discovered I actu-ally liked the peppery taste of arugula. In the grocery store I found myself looking at the salad dressings and decided I didn't want the pretentious organic stuff. I was pining for nostalgia: French dressing, Thousand Island, and Catalina. I didn't care about the calories because everything settles in the midsection anyways.

Over the years (yes, years) the cravings change and take you by surprise every time. The latest one to catch me off-guard was my compulsion to have Frank's hot sauce in the house. For four days of uncontrollable will, I really did put that shit on everything.

TEN

MY FIRST HOT FLASH

I was sitting at the kitchen table with my husband and his boss, who had flown in from Toronto the day before. Dinner was almost ready and the house was filled with the smell of prime rib roasting in the oven. We were nibbling on pâté and Brie and crackers, talking about camping, travel, and anything not related to work. My husband is fortunate to have a great relationship with his boss. They worked together at another company in the same relationship. He's been to our house several times for dinner, most notably once when my mother was visiting us in Calgary. She turned to him and said, "Now that you're over 50, have you had a prostate exam?" As we've already established, she is not a medical expert, nor does she have any training in that area. What she has is a remarkable capacity to let things fall unfiltered out of her mouth. After that kind of conversation, it's safe to say my husband felt confident nothing he could ever say to his boss would be uncomfortable.

This time, the three of us had wine glasses in front of us and Jeff had just poured each of us some red. After we toasted, I put my nose to the rim and sniffed. I was really looking forward to that feeling of the first sip. I don't drink often, but I know the merits of a much-needed glass of wine. I tilted the glass to my lips and let the wine fill my mouth. It was perfect. As the three of us sat and chatted, I continued to drink my wine. I was almost done the first glass when Jeff topped me up.

I was about to bring the glass to my mouth when I suddenly felt like something was very wrong. My head swam. A ripple went through my head from the base of my skull, over the back of my head to my forehead and my eyes lost focus. It felt like my eyeballs were bouncing around in their sockets like googly eyes. Before I could process what had happened, the weirdness stopped. I glanced at Jeff and his boss, but whatever I had just experienced went unnoticed by either of them. I held my wine in front of me, wondering if I should stop drinking. Surely the full glass of wine had simply gone directly to my head.

I had little more than a minute of normalcy before the next wave started. This one started in my upper abdomen. A bloom of heat, just below the bra line. It built as it travelled up my sternum. When it hit my neck, I lost my breath and felt squeezing in my chest. Without a word, I pushed my chair back and went upstairs to the master bathroom. I didn't want to interrupt the conversation by having a heart attack in the kitchen.

I leaned over the sink, my hands gripping the sides. Was I dying?

A band of sweat appeared across my forehead. My face was melting from the inside, but my skin only showed the slightest shade of red. I didn't look like I was dying; I looked embarrassed about dying.

My pulse was racing. I couldn't catch my breath. My

tongue felt too big for my mouth. My armpits went from dry to dripping instantly. The same happened under my breasts. *This must be what internal combustion feels like,* I thought. *Or heart failure.*

Not knowing what else to do, I turned on the water, letting it run cold. I cupped my hands under the faucet and leaned over to calm the heat by soaking my whole face in the palm of my hands. But before I could submerge myself completely, everything was back to normal. It was like a switch was turned off. There was no gradual cooling down, no need to sit down and take deep breaths. The fires of hell within had extinguished themselves and I was back in my right mind. Not today, Satan.

I wiped the sweat from my forehead, applied a swoosh of deodorant, and flushed the toilet, just in case the men downstairs were wondering where I was.

They weren't. They were absorbed in the crackling hunk of meat my husband had taken out of the oven and was wrapping to rest. I set the table in the dining room, plated the roasted potatoes, and tossed the salad like nothing at all had happened. I glanced at my phone charging on the kitchen counter, desperately wanting to look up the symptoms of a heart attack, but also not wanting to be rude. I was alive for now. Google wasn't going to change that.

I picked up my wine glass to take a sip, then put it back down. Whatever was wrong with me, wine was probably not going to help.

The words of their conversation were background noise to the humming in my head. I was sitting uncomfortably on the kitchen chair, hoping that whatever had just happened would not repeat itself. As I watched the steam rise from the freshly cut prime rib, two words popped into my brain: HOT FLASH.

As soon as I acknowledged them, I knew they were the truth. I wasn't suffering from angina or knocking at death's door. I was transitioning from perimenopause into menopausal territory. Like every woman, I had heard the tales of spontaneous sweating and dizzying heat from my mother and her friends. I only had one friend my age who had made it through to menopause already, and she functioned as my early warning system. I would ask about a symptom, she would nod and share her own experience. But to hear the seniors tell it, it was an excruciating process involving daily changing and washing of sheets, an embarrassing inability to remember anything, and a prolapsed uterus and vagina.

It turns out hot flashes come with their own special sauce of crazy.

"I was dying of heat," Christine told me, "so I had the air conditioning blasting as high as I could turn it. The kids kept saying the house was freezing and had blankets on them and warmer clothes. I kept thinking the A/C was broken because I was sweating horribly. I was on the phone with my husband telling him the A/C was broken. He told me to go to the furnace room and check it from there. Well, I get down to the furnace room and there was a full thick layer of ice on the pipes. I realized later that I was going through my first hot flash." Christine sent me a picture of the insulated copper pipes enrobed in a thick layer of ice. I haven't seen ice that compressed since 1978 when we defrosted years of accumulation in our freezer.

"Babe, I think I had my first hot flash today," I told Jeff that night as we settled into bed.

I lay there, feeling a different kind of heat. This time it

was more uncomfortable than life-threatening. I kicked the covers off and fanned my face with my hands.

"Great," he mumbled.

"What does that mean?" I asked, feeling indignant.

"Nothing. It doesn't mean anything. I'm sorry I said anything."

"It's not like I can control it," I huffed.

"I know. It's just... it's — "

"It's just what?"

"Okay, don't get mad, but this has been going on for years already."

Four years, at this point.

"I thought you were already having hot flashes. It's like sleeping beside a furnace sometimes."

I laughed because it was true. I have always run hot.

"This was different, though," I explained. "I thought my insides were melting."

"Sounds terrible. Just tell me what you need from me."

Hide the knives, I wanted to say. *Stop chewing so loud. Quit channel surfing and I might not set your leg hair on fire.*

"Thanks," I muttered to his back. He had already turned over, drifting off to sleep while I lay there, feeling the sweat build in every crevice.

ELEVEN

THE VAG

I f you are at all uncomfortable with too much information, skip this chapter. I'm going to be blunt about what happens with the vagina during peri-menopause and menopause. I'm not going to get medical because I am not a doctor. I will say this: if at any time you think something is very wrong "down there," suck up the embarrassment and ask your doctor about it. The last thing you want to do is wait it out. Ovarian cancer is a very serious thing, as is uterine cancer. Obviously, all cancer is a very serious thing, and your menopausal mind will immediately go there and you will think about mortality a lot. You will also think about your female anatomy and what is happening with your vagina. As we age, the vag does too. Some weird things start showing up — fibroids, fistulas, and fluids.

Buckle up, bitches. We're going in.

The things that happen to the vagina during peri-menopause are nothing you are going to discuss at wing night. You're not going to dip your saucy hot wing into blue cheese dressing and be triggered to bring up what those things have in common with your vag. If you are lucky, you'll have one girlfriend who is not shy about talking about the discharge, smells, and sensations she is experiencing. For now, you've got me.

Just when you think you are comfortable with your vagina, everything starts to go awry. For me, this meant copious discharge started flowing, indicating a period was coming. This was an important development, since the further I went into perimenopause, the less reliable my cycle became. This clear and odourless discharge was more of a nuisance than something to worry about. My drawer in the bathroom held a variety of feminine products: tampons, panty liners, vaginal wipes for when I'm just not feeling fresh, and a yeast infection treatment kit because sometimes the discharge is suspiciously thick and clumpy.

While I'm not going to invite you to find a mirror to examine yourself, you need to be extremely aware of what is not normal for you. My vagina functioned without any surprises until after I had my two kids. Then it started working a bit differently, but my gynecologist assured me there was nothing abnormal. As my perimenopause was coming to a close, I reverted to 12-year-old me who was grossed out, embarrassed, uncomfortable, and unfamiliar with that space between her legs. Menopause ages you backwards but not in the good way that face creams promise.

At some point during my during my journey, my vagina and my discharge started to smell horrible. It was mortifying to me. I thought the smell lingered after I went to the bathroom, like asparagus pee, but musky and sour. The first time the odour wafted up from the toilet bowl, I figured a yeast infection was the cause. I waited a day or two before I decided to use the kit. As anyone who has a vagina will tell you, periodic odours are not unusual. But the next day, and the day after that, the smell did not wane. Adding the yeast infection treatment to the mix made a god-awful mess. I apologize for this, but the stuff coming out of my vagina was reminiscent of fondue made with curdled Limburger cheese. Needless to say, sex was off the table for a bit. All I could say to my husband was ,"There is something going crazy with my vagina." When I saw the smirk on his face, I quickly added, "and not in a good way."

As if the punishment of a weepy, stinky vagina isn't enough, menopause can bring with it fistulas and fibroids. As the vaginal wall weakens, it's possible for a hole — a fistula — to open up inside. Mine came on the heels of a diverticular abscess, providing a convenient way for the infection to get out of my body. It is as disgusting as it sounds. Sex was off the table again and this time, I was more direct with Jeff.

"Pus is coming out of my vagina." No further comment required.

While I never experienced fibroids, some friends have had issues with them. Fibroids can grow anywhere in or on our reproductive system. These growths tend to be painful, but are usually non-cancerous. Someone I know had extremely painful fibroids on her uterus and had surgery to remove them. She had her uterus and ovaries removed as well, going from a single hot flash to the other side of menopause in about three hours. This is not what every woman will experience, but it's a worst-case scenario.

As your vagina changes, so does your relationship with it. I developed a familiarity with all its bumps, sensations, and textures. You will too. Some days, you may find your vagina is drier than usual and sex may be painful because your natural lubricant is no longer present. Sometimes you'll be itchy. Vaginal wipes helped me with that. A woman in my circle found a growth on the inside of her labia when she went to scratch. At age 51, she felt comfortable enough to share this with me with all the casualness and excitement of telling me about an amazing handbag she found at Marshalls.

"So scratching the itch is like a vaginal self-exam," I said to her.

"And just as satisfying." She winked at me.

Every woman will have a completely different experience "down there." Pay attention. Be upfront with your spouse. Check with your doctor if your gut is telling you this is something more than just menopause. You will only feel foolish if you don't do anything about it and it turns out to be something serious.

TWELVE

SEXUAL HEALING

"You know what's wonderful about sex? It's free and it feels good."

One of my best friends shared this nugget with me decades ago. It's an accurate statement.

Before perimenopause started, I'd never really given deep thought to my sex life. I took it for granted that everything was working as it should. I had a healthy sex drive, with a realistic mix of attentive and inconsiderate partners. In my twenties and thirties, sex evolved from being a distraction to being an important part of an intimate relationship. By the time I was near the end of my perimenopause, sex had presented some interesting challenges.

For some women, the libido can turn on and gush like Niagara Falls; for others it can go as dark as a continental power outage. I have a friend who candidly shared with me that she would call her husband to come home from work over lunch to have quick, extremely satisfying sex.

"Best sex since my dirty thirties," she said with a giggle.

With apologies to Jeff, my experience was nothing like

that. My sex spigot was firmly in the off position, despite my desire to have it to go the other way.

Jeff and I had once had a very healthy sex life. The disinterest in sex wove itself into my psyche. I didn't wake up one day and decide I didn't want any, it just kind of faded out of our lives. Life was exhausting. We were on a hamster wheel of kids-work-home-chores-errands-obligations and we couldn't see where to get off (sorry, not sorry). Our sex drives were suddenly way out of sync. I'd move over and start caressing Jeff's chest and he would wrap his arm around me, but that would be it.

"Are you coming on to me?" he'd ask.

"Maybe," I'd say, wrapping myself in a protective layer of non-commitment.

"I'd love to, but I'm so tired and I have a migraine starting."

And that was the end of that. I'd turn away from him, feeling spurned but somewhat relieved that I, too, could go to sleep.

Some nights, Jeff would reach out to me and I would let him play, but there was nothing stirring within me. His touch felt like a cozy, weighted blanket, and I was just as responsive to his fingers as I would be to the fleece. It felt nice and I didn't have to engage. Telling your husband he reminds you of something that shows up for sale in your Facebook feed is not conducive to satisfying orgasms. The worst part of all of this was that I didn't care.

There were nights I would turn away with relief and nights where I would want to cry, feeling rejected. Perimenopause does a fantastic job of fucking with your emotions. Not only are you not in control of how you feel, your emotions are now contained inside a cocktail shaker. At any given moment, your feels will be a jumbled mess —

shaken, not stirred — and you'll have no idea which one will pour out first. The chaos churned within me. The desire to make out with my husband was coupled with the rage of knowing the laundry still sat unfolded in the basket in the laundry room. The abundant love I felt for my husband was overshadowed by the fear that I could have a heart attack in my sleep. The memory of our healthy sex life was washed away by the incessant chatter in my brain about how I am a bad wife: unloving, uncaring, and not putting out.

For the better part of three years, sex became an extremely occasional activity. As my middle filled out and I struggled to lose any weight, I felt less and less attractive. If ever in my life I felt I was walking around with a black cloud over my head, it was during this period in my life. I wondered if Jeff found me unattractive or if he was struggling with something too. He is always the stoic one, my loving husband, the perfect cliché of a strong man. Even if he was feeling unloved, or uncomfortable, or unhappy, he would never tell me. I get to go through my things first. I get to be moody and irrational. I was allowed to be an ogre and he would still show me he loved me. That alone should have been a turn on.

I knew, without a doubt, that our marriage could survive this blackout because as my libido withered, my love for my husband grew. Despite the occasional desire to push him out of the moving car, I could look at my husband sitting on the couch and feel an enormous abundance of love fill me. It really is a physical sensation: a bubble of joy that starts in the stomach and moves its way to warm my heart. It's not gas or a hot flash; it's pure love. Whenever I felt like this, I knew that even if we never had sex again, we would be okay.

"We talk about the fact that we should," Carrie said

about her sex life with her husband, "and sometimes we do. But it's us both making an effort versus being driven by desire. Desire lives more in my memories of what was versus what I want to do today."

I know exactly how she feels. When Jeff and I are both invested in sex, it's rewarding, satisfying, and strengthens our bond. After, as we lay in bed drifting off to sleep, we wonder aloud why we don't do this more, because, yes, it's free and it feels good.

I carry immense guilt about my lacking libido. I have to acknowledge that there is nothing I can do without medication. That is not a route I am ready to take yet. I'll wait until the kids have moved out of the house and Jeff and I can really take advantage of the benefits.

A woman I know, Janis, had a hysterectomy when she was 34 and had, she said, "zero indication that my body was going through 'the change'. But let's talk about the lack of sex drive. The way I described it to my doctor was if sex were a car. I'm in Calgary (physical me), my car is parked in Florida (the idea of sex) and my keys are in New Zealand (libido). How in the world did I get so far removed from it? His response was, 'Well, at least you know where the keys are.'"

There is hope, though. Just as my friend's afternoon delights waned, so has my flickering of desire started to re-emerge. Once I was fully menopausal, I began to realize that the tingling in my labia wasn't just me needing to pee. It was the renewed flow of blood to my vag. With this slow reawakening came erotic dreams in which my husband and I were restored to our former sexual glory. In my dreams, we didn't care where or when or who was in the room, we just wanted to make love all the time. It was liberating and exciting.

Every single time, I woke up from these sexy dreams feeling warm and fuzzy and ready for some action. I would lie there, on my back with my eyes still closed, holding on to the fading images of the two of us, sweaty and glowing and happy. I would turn my head to my husband, wondering if I should wake him up or let him get his much-needed sleep. In that split second, the eros dimmed, my lady parts lost their heat, and my head filled with all the things I needed to get done that day. My libido had switched on, then off. A pit of sadness formed in my abdomen, lamenting the missed opportunity. I should have jumped him when I had the chance.

As in athletics, firefighting, and neurosurgery, seconds matter in the menopausal world. The menopausal brain can process a coherent thought and lose all logic in the space of two seconds. If you've ever found yourself talking on your smartphone and then searching for that same smartphone to look up something, welcome to the menopausal club. In those precious seconds I spent lying in bed, I squeezed my eyes tighter, hoping to bring back some of that loving feeling, but the only thing I manifested was the desperate urge to empty my bladder. Thanks a lot, menopause.

THIRTEEN

YOU NEVER LISTEN TO ME

J eff really is the best husband I've ever had. He likes
to joke that since my first husband turned out to be
gay with a propensity toward seedy bathhouses, "it
gives me a wide window of fucking up to work
with."

My husband is supportive of everything I've ever tried
to do. He was onboard when we decided it made sense for
me to stay home and raise the boys. He's never complained
about my housecleaning even though he knows it isn't a
failure in ability but an absence of will. When I launched
my business, Digital Shoebox, he encouraged me from the
start, and kept quiet for many years as I struggled to turn it
into something more than a way to pass time and fund my
frozen coffee addiction. He eats everything I put in front of
him, even after we discovered he is the better cook and I am
the skilled baker. He is my cheerleader, my champion, and
the yang to my mid-life, menopausal, unreliable yin.

Most days I can confidently say we have a stable relationship. Like any married couple, we have our fights. Not
really big blowouts, but disagreements where one of us lets

it rip while the other gets pouty and silent. I bounce back from my anger faster than Jeff does; he can stew for a whole day about something I said, did, didn't do, or completely forgot.

It's that last bit that is important here: "completely forgot." It took more than a year for me to clue in that my brain was working differently in perimenopause. It wasn't the first time my mind had decided to lower its capacity for smartness. After the boys were born, I had mommy brain. I was tired, lonely, and losing my mind pushing trains around a track while watching endless episodes of *Thomas the Tank Engine*. (I maintain the boys learned their colours and numbers from the engines at Tidmouth Sheds. As they started to talk, they had slight British accents.) Like every mom with littles at home, I was easily distracted, confused, and lost track of time. Most days, however, I was able to get dinner on the table and remember to take a shower. Once those hormones cleared, I was restored to my former glory: I could focus, finish my sentences, and have an adult conversation. That didn't last long.

By the time the boys hit their teen years, my brain chemistry was changing without my knowledge. At first it was small things like looking for keys while they were in my hand or putting the milk in the pantry and the coffee in the dishwasher. As time marched on, I would stop in the middle of the room, completely unaware of what I had come in for. Sadly, this happened mostly in the kitchen, where the only assumption I could make was that I came in for something to eat. I attribute my greatest weight gain to grazing on crackers when I really needed to get a stamp from the junk drawer. My 15-year-old helpfully pointed out my memory failures.

"Look what I found at the thrift store!" I exclaimed with glee one afternoon as I showed him a book I purchased.

"Umm, Mom, didn't you already read that?"

I shook my head. "Nope. It's been on my list for a few years though."

"Mom, I'm sure you read that book, like, six months ago. You got it at the library."

I picked up the book and opened up to the first page, reading a few sentences, but there was no hint of familiarity.

I shook my head again.

"I don't think I read it."

"Maybe you should check that app where you keep track of all your books."

In a prideful effort to prove that I was right, I did just that. I opened up Goodreads and searched my books for the title. I stared at the screen and then forced out a laugh. I didn't want my kid to think his mother had really lost her shit.

"You're right," I acknowledged. "I did read this already. I guess I read so many books I lose track sometimes." I shrugged and smiled. He rolled his eyes then walked off.

I had read the book almost two years ago. It took less than 730 days for the text to be completely wiped from my mind. Still, I had bought the book and was now obligated to read it again. It took about 80 pages for things to become familiar. I could have stopped reading, but I'd invested $4.99 in this book and I was going to finish it. Again.

I should have been alarmed that I had such a blank spot in my memory, but my addled menopausal brain protected me. I would have conversations with Jeff where we'd make decisions about things and I would have no recollection of any of it. I could sit at the dinner table and give him my full attention and within a week, I would have completely forgotten every single word. I wish I could blame looking at my phone while he spoke and say my attention was diverted, but that wasn't the case.

"You never listen to me!" he exclaimed one evening, exasperated that I had forgotten yet another conversation.

I stared at him from my seat on the couch with nothing to say. I had no defence. I was wrapped in my own thoughts, trying desperately to bring back any shred of memory of the conversation he was referring to.

"I do listen," I finally said. "But for some reason, I can't remember the conversation. I have zero recollection that we had any words about this. At all."

He looked at me like I was crazy, a justified reaction.

"I don't doubt we talked about this," I said. "What room were we in when we had this discussion?"

"Why does that matter?" he asked.

"It might jog my memory," I explained.

"We were right here, in the living room."

I looked around the room, trying to imagine the original conversation. Still, there was nothing. Not a shred of déjà vu. I could understand his frustration because it mirrored my own. How many conversations have I had that were completely wiped from my memory?

Here's where I should have been afraid. Knowing I may have made promises I forgot about or committed to things I couldn't recall should have worried me. I may not have known how many conversations I'd forgotten, but I did know this had nothing to do with dementia or Alzheimer's. This was a blip caused by hormones changing my chemistry. For once in my life, I didn't feel the need to consult

Dr. Google in search of a condition that matched my list of symptoms. I knew in my gut that this was menopause.

"I'm sorry hun, but I don't remember any of this. I *am* listening to you. I hear you. My brain just wipes it from my memory. I am not arguing that we had these conversations. I'm just asking you not to get mad because I can't remember. This isn't me not paying attention, this is my brain being controlled by menopause."

As my memory reservoir failed, I found I was gaslighting myself. I was filled with so much doubt about what conversations really happened. I'd replay entire conversations I thought happened, but never actually did. I'd scrape my memory banks for remnants of conversations that had in fact happened. It's frightening to not be able to separate the actual from the imagined.

Fortunately, a conscious awareness came with the confusion. I knew to be cognizant of what was happening. When I became aware of a memory lapse, I didn't have to freak out. "It's just menopause" became my mantra. I shrugged off my vacant mind as a menopausal symptom, but made a mental note to keep track of any further incidents. This turned out to be a futile exercise, though. Mental notes flutter away as quickly as I make them in my failing menopausal mind.

I had a frightening lapse when I was driving to a familiar destination. I blanked and forgot how to get to a strip mall I had visited more than 20 times in the past five years. I had to pull over to the shoulder, take some deep breaths, and live in that fear for a few moments. How could I have no recollection of where to go? I sat in the car, looking out the windshield, then my side windows, then my rear-view mirror trying to get my bearings. For a few terrifying moments, I had no idea which direction I was facing.

When I was out of panic mode, I was able to set my GPS to take me where I needed to go. It was a horrible feeling, being completely lost like that, and I couldn't shake it off for the rest of the day. So far, that incident has not been repeated, but it has left me feeling haunted and afraid that it could happen again.

FOURTEEN

MALE MENOPAUSE

This page intentionally left blank.

FIFTEEN

FRIENDSHIPS

Friendships haven't always come easy to me, so when I find the good ones, I tend to hold them close. I'm still in contact with a few of my childhood friends and one or two of my high school chums. I find it amusing to watch my longtime friends evolve into adults with spouses and kids, so far removed from the hair-teasing, lip-glossing, gossip-spreading teenagers we used to be. It's a privilege to have friends for that long. You'd think we would be able to share anything, having popped zits together at sleepovers, but when it comes to menopause, we clam up. Women share tons of information about pregnancy through forums and on social media where strangers share unsolicited advice. But when we start our perimenopausal journey, we fall silent. It's fascinating that these two huge hormonal shifts and life changes are so differently considered.

Adult friendships are a whole other beast. Since we are not forced together every day in school, making new friends is more complicated. I used to have university friends — optimists and barflies — whom I spent hours with during the four years of my undergrad. But after graduation, we all floated on to the next parts of life and I've barely seen them since.

After university I had my work friends. We occasionally hung out at lunch or hit the pub on Fridays after work. There always seems to be an arms-length distance from work colleagues. Like high school, little cliques tend to form. The line between those who work hard and those who hardly work is clearly marked. My colleagues came and went and moved on to better jobs, or worse, became my boss.

When I had kids, my world became populated with mom friends, most of who had kids in the same age range as mine. We bitched and moaned and laughed and cried and bonded over explosive poops, spit-up mashed peaches that landed in our mouths, and mouth-wide-open slobbery kisses we wouldn't trade for anything in this world. Despite all the moves across the country, my mommy friends are the ones that I still have to this day. We are tied together through the bodily fluids of our children and many cups of coffee spiked with Baileys Irish Cream. We are all moving together through the various milestones — our own as well as those of our offspring — and I consider many of them to be my best friends. Our children are now teenagers and we've all kept in touch since our kids were a year or two old. These women have been my lifeline and have filled my social calendar with dinner clubs, books clubs, and ladies' week-ends away without the kids. Nothing solidifies a friendship like a night in a cabin in the Rockies drinking copious amounts of wine and swapping labour stories.

It was heartbreaking when I left these friends behind as we moved from Calgary, Alberta, to Surrey, British Columbia. Jeff was travelling extensively for work. I had landed in a community where I knew nobody and had no idea what resources were available to me, a mom with a three-year-old and a four-year-old. I didn't know it at the time, but my emotional state was being influenced by the very early stages of perimenopause, adding a whole new level of anxiety to my ability to make friends.

We moved into our house on a swampy, humid day in August and the first neighbour I met in the back lane driveway greeted us with this:

"So, you're from Alberta, huh?" he said, pointing his chin toward the license plate on my mini-van. "Got tired of making all that money?"

I gave the speaker a thin-lipped smile and tossed back my secret weapon: feigned stupidity.

"What do you mean?" I asked, giving him the blankest stare I could.

There was a satisfying moment of awkwardness before he sputtered out, "Umm, I meant, like, umm, you know, the oil and gas money. It's booming out there, right?"

"I guess," I shrugged. And I just left it at that. It was a weird moment for me. Being the new kid on the block, I should have been polite and accommodating. This was my opportunity to start making friends. As I walked back into my house to start unpacking boxes, a feeling of delight washed over me. For the first time in my life, instead of silently absorbing someone else's rude behaviour, I pushed back without being defensive. It might have been fatigue that made me react that way, or maybe it was the first inkling of age-related self-confidence that I'd heard emerges in our forties. On this particular day there was no sign of the people-pleasing woman I'd become who would have been horrified over the thought of making someone feel uncomfortable. The voices in my head would have been trying to figure out a way to make amends so I could make friends. But on that day, I didn't care if they liked me. I wasn't the assuming asshole in this situation.

I stood in my kitchen, surrounded by boxes stacked four high and felt good about deciding these were not the kind of people with whom I wanted to be friends. This was the first step in identifying that I had the power to choose whose company I kept. I was finally acting like a confident adult. Over the next three years, I never got close to any of the people with whom we shared the lane. I was polite and courteous, but something in my perimenopausal gut told me to trust my first impression.

My suspicions were confirmed one early spring weekday evening when I sat quietly in my backyard, enjoying a break in the rain and sipping a hot cup of tea. The boys were in the house, thoroughly absorbed by a video and I took a mommy moment to breathe. My peace was broken when I heard some of my neighbours pulling chairs into the lane and opening a bottle of wine to share. I was happy to eavesdrop on their chatter. I wasn't surprised when one of them started talking about me and making fun of the "size of that ass." I smiled to myself, secure in the knowledge that I made the right choice in not putting any effort into being friends with these people. They will always be petty and jealous and mean. Some people never get past the high school mentality.

As I listened to their banter, I made the decision to better curate my friendships. I was no longer going to put up with any bullshit. If my jackass meter was beeping madly when we first met, that was going to be my measure. The words of Maya Angelou came to mind. "When people show you who they are, believe them." The mindset shift was liberating. Over the next decade, friends would come and go. As we moved from British Columbia to Ontario and then back to Alberta, I made friends who acted as my support until I found my footing in the new-to-me neighbourhood. Then, as time passed, I would discover I had little in common with my new friend and I would quietly drift away. I let go of the need to hang on to friends who made me feel like garbage. I stopped calling the friends who made me work overtime to be their friend. I accepted the quirks and qualms of the friends who were good people and worth keeping around.

As I moved closer to being fully menopausal, I started to examine my own behaviour in my friendships. I struggled to recognize when my expectations were unreasonable. When my hormones were on full alert (i.e. in completely crazy mode), I was ready to shut myself off from the world, unfriend everyone, and be done with socializing. When I thought about my own role in friendships, I realized I had a tendency to place my friends under deeper scrutiny than I was willing to put on myself. My husband often talked me off the ledge of rage and betrayal. He would tell me I have two choices: I could end the friendship or I could just accept that everyone has imperfections. And the right to make their own decisions about things that impact me in no way at all. It pissed me off that he was right. I would vacillate between being angry at a friend for being self-absorbed when I needed her support and being touched to the core by the simple gesture of her dropping a book off at my house.

Once I reached the other side of menopause and passed my 50th birthday, my friendships, and how I managed them, matured. I dumped fair-weather friends. I unfollowed the drama llamas on Facebook. I recognized who were my true friends and which people were still around to serve my needs. This was a surprise revelation: it was okay for me to keep in touch with someone just because they filled a temporary gap in my life, as many did when we moved to a new neighbourhood. At this stage in my life, I know it's okay to let someone go when the relationship doesn't feel right anymore. I do my best not to be hurtful to others, but I'm sure someone on the other end of the friendship string is wondering why they are still friends with me. If they choose to cut me loose, I'm okay with that. I won't waste any time in self-reflection, wondering where the friendship went wrong. I won't try to salvage a relationship that served to only make me angry, bitter, or heartbroken.

In a fit of nostalgia, I've reached out to a few friends from the past. It should have come as no surprise that my genial, laid-back childhood friend became the hands-off, let-children-be-who-they-are kind of mom. Those who were kind when we were kids are still kind today. I've welcomed back the smart, ambitious ones who may have stepped on people on their climb to the top then gained some valuable humility on the way back down. The point is I'm now choosing who I welcome into my circle, who gets shut out, and who gets kicked off Dana Island.

The most important lesson I learned about friendships during my menopausal journey is to appreciate the gifts, good and bad, that others bring into your life. A gift could be a sense of awareness about yourself. It may be recognizing the mad talent of some of your friends and just enjoying what they create. Maybe they're around to teach you something, enlighten you, or change the way you think. Many friends will come and go throughout our lifetimes. The ones you keep are those who can make you laugh while calling you a dickhead at the same time.

SIXTEEN

SLEEP AND LACK THEREOF

F*uck. Not again. Why is this happening? Okay, just breathe. Deep breath in, slow breath out. Focus on the breath. Breathe in calm, breathe out noise. Breathe in peace, breathe out turmoil. Focus on the breathing. Stop thinking about other — What if I empty the linen closet and re-organize it? Do we really need all those ratty towels? Why am I keeping the sheets for bed sizes we no longer have? Fuck. Here we go again. Breathe in...*

If you are in perimenopause, y'all have had this kind of conversation in your head at roughly 2:37 a.m. You got up to pee, and when you got back into bed, the chatter in your brain just wouldn't stop. If you haven't yet experienced this new, disruptive sleep pattern, take my advice and just pee the bed. Don't get out of that warm cocoon you're in, because as soon as you do, you're doomed. You'll spend the next one-and-a-half to two hours trying to fall back asleep. At best you'll hover somewhere between slightly asleep and raging brain activity.

Sleep during this stage of life is plagued with an assortment of inconveniences. Some mornings, you'll wake up feeling like you are in a swamp, with sheets that are wet with sweat and now need to be washed. Sometimes, it's just your head that is sweating, and while your hair is stuck like soaked fur to the back of your neck, your legs are freezing. The back of your head will get so itchy, you'll wonder if you have lice, then spend the next 40 minutes figuring out how you got it and calculating how many loads of laundry you'll have to do until your brain suddenly switches to ruminating on the history of lice and how it seems unfair for them to be associated with dirtiness when they're really as pervasive as the common cold.

Yes, my friends, this is your brain on perimenopause.

When you're not busy considering the injustices wrought upon the innocent louse, your perimenopausal brain will fill the empty hours when you cannot sleep with a list of irrational fears, most of which are tied to your newly simmering generalized anxiety. These night fears will cover a wide range of topics and life events, from things you will almost never encounter to the daily minutiae. For example:

- Did I pay the credit card bill on time?
- Did I pay the right amount?
- Did I even see the bill in the mail?
- Is the fridge in the garage open?
- Is my husband breathing? (Look over to confirm that he is, just in case.)
- If I were snorkelling in Australia and got stung by a jellyfish, would it leave a scar?
- What do I need to do to run for government office?
- How can I grow my business?
- Does the bank watch all our transactions and

know that we have $6.79 in our chequing
account?

- How many days out of the year does it rain in
Singapore?
- Why does my hair feel
thicker/thinner/drier/greasier today?

Every single thought is random. They flit in and out of
my brain faster than a meerkat in its hidden hole. It should
be noted that I never come up with any answers to these
questions. It's all just a big rhetorical game my mind plays
in order to prevent me from getting what I really crave: a
decent night's sleep.

Night after night, I found myself panicking, pondering,
and pandering. I'd try to make a deal with my brain. *Please
just let me get a couple more hours' sleep and I'll feed you
salad all day. Come on. If you stop right now, later today I'll
let you get lost in a really good book.* I tried a more
belligerent approach: *Fuck you. I'm just going to lie here
until the alarm goes off. I'm going to count the bumps in the
popcorn ceiling. I'm going to mindlessly drift off to sleep and
you can't do anything to stop me.*

There was no clear response from my brain, but I am
pretty sure I heard a low-throated snigger, a "heh heh heh"
that was layered with scorn and the knowledge that comes
with imminent victory. *There will be no more sleep for you
tonight, my pretty.*

Night after night, this terrible game plays out. The
wicked witch of menopausal unrest takes control. If I get
more than five hours of uninterrupted sleep, it is a gift she
has bestowed on me. I have tried drinking an herbal nighttime tea, and while that helps me fall asleep, it also makes
me have to go pee and sends me right back into the

insomnia loop. I've taken melatonin with good results, but the tiny herbal supplements are not always reliable against the hormonal battle that is taking place inside my body. In my attempts to fall back asleep, I have visualized waves rolling onto the beach or a misty fog rolling into the mountains and I have imagined feeling the gentle caress of ferns in a moonlit forest. These nighttime exercises have only served to force me out of bed to the bathroom, lead my brain to a 90-degree turn from a pastoral setting to the set of a horror film, and make me so itchy I scratch imaginary rashes.

What's the moral of this story? Know this is coming, try to deal with it, but give in. Take naps if there is ever an opportunity. Do your best not to wake your partner, because two cranky people — one of whom is menopausal — will make for inflammatory conversations. Accept that there will be nights when you surprise yourself by sleeping through the night and nights when you will lie in bed trying to summon the sleep genie who will ultimately lead you into a silent sing-along in your head of the greatest hits from Disney movies. *You ain't never had a friend like me.*

SEVENTEEN

CRANKY IS MY DEFAULT

S omewhere on the road between perimenopause and menopause, I settled into what I call my hostile period. For the better part of a year, cranky was my default setting. Hormones gave me the green light to be an absolute sobbing mess and then pivot to a raging asshole.

While everything made me cranky, some things progressed to also make me either angry or disgusted:

- the inequity of pricing at the dry cleaner's (men's shirts are less expensive to dry clean than women's blouses, even though most men's shirts need to be starched and pressed!)
- friends who post filtered photos on social media when I know they don't *ever* look like that
- the sight of blood seeping onto the cutting board from a freshly roasted prime rib
- any kind of grammatical error

It didn't take much to turn me from a Julie Andrews to a Joan Crawford.

I was in crank mode for a very long time. I would wake up with a pit of resentment in my stomach. I looked in the mirror and was exasperated by the appearance of new wrinkles. I hated the way my hair looked and how my clothes fit. The chaos in the linen closet would distract me for days until, in a fit of unreasonable aggravation, I would pull everything out into a massive pile on the floor and spend the better part of an hour deciding what needed to go. When my husband showed any kind of sentimental attachment to anything to do with our children, I rolled my eyes and questioned his motives.

"It's probably time we updated these photos," I said, pointing to the school photos in our bedroom.

"Why?" he asked. "I like these."

"Yeah, but they're four years old."

"So?"

"So, it's time to move on. Let them go, Jeff. Let's not turn into those parents who keep a wall of outdated photos on display. We've got more recent pictures that are better."

"No. I like these ones and I want them to stay."

I glared at him, willing him to change his mind, but he walked away from me before I could say another word. I looked at the photos, deciding whether he would notice if I changed them. I vacillated for a moment, wondering if I even cared what he thought. I weighed the option of just doing whatever I wanted versus sustaining a happy marriage. I stared at those dated photos, lost in the baby-toothed grins and absorbed by the happiness in their eyes. My heart filled with such love for my boys, then on the verge of becoming teenagers. While reflective of their young innocence, it was time for the photos to go. I headed downstairs to sift through the photos on my computer and got lost in memories of the past year. I had a couple of photos in mind, but when I couldn't find them in the latest dated folder, I headed over to Facebook to browse my photos there, hoping to pinpoint the correct year the photos were taken. I spent the better part of an hour deleting old albums, clicking on photos to see what status update I posted with them, and then completely forgot about my original mission. The elementary school photos of the boys are still hanging, three years after our conversation. I didn't give in, I got distracted.

The whole situation is exacerbated by the natural progression to middle age. As I settled into my later forties, an awareness of who I am and how I perceive the world cemented itself in my consciousness. I was now a cranky perimenopausal woman who didn't give a crap what other people thought.

Carrie recalled for me the "crankenators" from her workplace when she was in her early thirties. These women were generally angry and dismissive and never seemed to be satisfied with anything.

"I thought this middle-aged person was an asshole," she said. "Now *I* am the asshole."

I had flashbacks of my younger days when I would party, get drunk, and say exactly what was on my mind. If you had stupid hair, I might have suggested you find a new hairdresser. If you were a bitch all the time, I'd ask you what was going on at home that made you so unhappy. If you were an egomaniacal pretty boy, I'd tell you to enjoy it because looks fade. I'd wake up the next morning, sometimes at home, sometimes not, with the knowledge that I had lost some friends, but found some new allies. That was high school and university though. Blurting out what's on my mind during middle age isn't so forgivable. I can understand why telling a friend it's time to ditch her slutty, low-cut blouses might be a dealbreaker. These days, I am more apt to just absorb what other people say and do and, for the most part, smile and keep my big mouth shut. It's not always easy.

I felt like I was living in a series of *Little Miss* books. On any given day, I would start out as Little Miss Sunshine, Little Miss Chatterbox, and Little Miss Fabulous. By dinner, I could be a whole lot of Little Miss Bossy, Little Miss Contrary, and Little Miss Scary. By bedtime, my family had avoided any further communication with me. I wasn't bothered by it all, for Little Miss Scatterbrain had already scrubbed my outbursts and crankiness from my mind.

As perimenopause turned into full-on menopause, I emerged with a new inner strength and comfort with what my personality was going to be like for the next little while. I didn't need to explain myself because no one was listening. Yet, every woman will walk this tenuous line at some point in her life. I pitied the 25-year-old with the 30-minute nighttime anti-aging regime who didn't know any better. I admired the tenacity of women in their early forties who struggled to hold on to their youth and trim waists and I smiled ruefully at their fruitless efforts. I had to allow my hormones the freedom to drive for a while and keep the saucy comments to myself. Menopause is not forgiving, but I am tougher than my hormones.

EIGHTEEN

ATTENTION SPAN

I could probably write this chapter in one sentence: in outlining the chapters for this book, I wrote "Attention Span" on the list twice. That sums up your perimenopausal brain's capacity for retaining information.

It's beyond frustrating to know you cannot hold on to information for very long. This lack of focus manifested itself around Year 4 of my seven-year perimenopausal journey. It's not a symptom that goes away, and I've always been a bit ditsy in that department. I cannot remember the birthdays of most of my friends, but the worst is that I cannot remember the birthday month of a friend of 35 years. The focus required to function in daily life has become more taxing than I care to admit. It's like my brain has 14 tabs open, all related to one another by the thinnest of threads. All it takes is for my dog to put her head on my knee while I'm working and I've lost the next two hours. I'll look at her cute face and realize she needs brushing, which leads to vacuuming the house, which leads to giving her a Milk-Bone because the noise stressed her out, which then leads to ordering more Milk-Bones and a webcam for one of the boys from Amazon.

It's always at times when I am trying my best to concentrate that my brain searches for a variety of tasks to pull me away. The tasks are usually the ones I procrastinate about: anything housekeeping related, picking up the dog poo from the yard, or restoring organization to the kitchen. Or my ever-loving husband suddenly wants to talk to me about buying stocks or sharing his dream for what he would do if we won the lottery.

The inability to rein in my lack of attention is not a symptom of adult ADHD. During this most hormonal phase of an adult woman's life (outside pregnancy and post-partum), the mind just wanders. Thoughts drift away like smoke in the wind. I have 40-plus years of memories, experiences, and emotions rolling around in there. They will force their way to the front of the line at the most inopportune moments. I was once heading to the kitchen to start making dinner and the phone rang. The setting sun was hitting my face in the right spot, so I headed outside, phone at my ear, to have my conversation. The sun felt warm, a blessed experience on this early fall day. I chatted with my childhood friend, laughed about life, and pined for our youth. Forty minutes later, when I was off the phone, I sat back and let the sun warm my skin. The breeze kicked up and I felt the promise of cooler days ahead and I realized I needed some new sweatshirts. It's an interesting development, since for the last six years, anything that covered more skin than necessary was shunned. In Year 2 of peri-menopause, in the midst of a sweaty, uncomfortable hot flash, I bagged all of my sweaters and long-sleeve shirts and dropped them at the thrift shop. I had no desire to replace the sweaters. This time, I wanted the soft cottony cuddle of a sweatshirt. I opened up the browser on my phone and started shopping, looking for deals. I found a site that had sweatshirts with cutesy sayings like "The mountains are calling and I must go," or "Talk to me after coffee," or "Bitch, please." I wanted sweatshirts that were more reflective of this stage of life with sayings like "This is your future," or "Error 404. Memory not found," or "Menopause lives here. Proceed with caution," but I had to settle for some cute pastel camo prints. Mission complete and I will have my sweatshirts in hand before the leaves are off the trees.

"Hello?" I heard Jeff call out from inside the house.

If he's home, it's well past six o'clock.

Fuck.

We will be ordering takeout tonight.

Let's play again.

I was writing a proposal for a client and suddenly I found myself examining an age spot on my forearm and wondering how long it's been there and if it's an age spot or melanoma and then I remembered the weird spot on my calf and wondered if that's the start of varicose veins. I immediately consulted Dr. Google, looking at images both benign and disgusting of various stages of skin cancer. I didn't have anything remotely similar, so I could rest easy. I opened Facebook and within two thumb scrolls, I was presented with an ad for age-spot reduction cream. I headed back to Google to read reviews, where I decided I don't need to spend $85 on 14 squirts of the magic serum and pulled my hand cream out of my purse because I noticed my skin was looking cracked. What was I doing before this?

Here's the summary: Imagine if Alice went down the rabbit hole and stopped at every twig on the way, then followed every twig to the next branch and by the time she was ready to find her way to the rabbit she was 50 years old and wondering why she thought she still could pull off the pinafore.

It's not all bad news in the attention span department. My wandering mind can just as easily get lost in the chirping of the birds in the trees or the rising sun bouncing off the waves of the ocean. I have stopped talking mid-sentence when low clouds hugging the mountains took my words away. I have also been gleefully distracted by my husband who wanders into my sightline as I write this, dressed handsomely in a T-shirt, underwear, and black knee socks.

There is no point fighting it. The brain is going to do what it wants to do, when it wants to do it and then it will shift when it finds a shiny, new object on which to focus. I have found it more rewarding to give in and accept this is the new way I have to do things. I've never fished, but I know what it looks like to reel in the line. I have to do that from time to time, but it's just as valuable to let your mind roam and take its own journey. Sure, you'll miss some deadlines or forget to cook dinner, and the laundry might sit in the washing machine for two days, but you might discover something amazing about yourself and the world when you veer off the path.

NINETEEN

BURIED, CRUSHED, AND ATTACKED
BY WOLVES

I *think I'm having a heart attack.*

I can't die right now. I haven't sent Jeff an email with all our passwords.

The kids cannot grow up with this loss.

Just take some deep breaths.

If I don't change some things, I'm not going to see the boys get married and I won't get to be a grandma.

These are the thoughts plaguing me at 3:11 a.m. Early in my perimenopause, I was not yet waking up to go to the bathroom or from some random dream or nightmare. I just woke up with a brain full of anxiety. During the daylight hours, it was business as usual for me with not a hint of the worries that kept me up. But most nights I would lie in bed unable to fall back asleep while my brain ran through its playlist of "Topics to Keep You Awake and Anxious."

My mortality was top of the list. Without warning, I would be wracked with fear about my impending death. I lay awake and imagined scenarios where I could die unexpectedly. Car accidents. Heart failure. Attacked by wolves while walking in the park. In my head, I mapped out a conversation with my husband where I tell him we should never put ourselves in a situation where, if something disastrous should happen, our children would be left parentless.

"Maybe we should start taking separate flights," I suggest in my mind.

He looks at me like I'm crazy and then concedes that we need to at least appoint a guardian. I'll reconsider and point out that it's good that we only ever go on vacations as a family because if the plane goes down, at least we are all together. Then he'll pedantically point out that we still need to appoint a guardian in case one of the boys survives while the rest of us perish. Oh, and we should also take care of getting our wills done. Then I glanced over at the clock and discovered this imaginary conversation took 16 minutes to build in my head, including revisions and alternate locations.

If I felt a twinge of new pain in my breast, I worried about breast cancer. If my poop came out skinny, I talked myself into believing I had rectal cancer. On more than one occasion, after I passed poop tinted with red, I sat for an extended period of time on the toilet, searching for the symptoms of stomach cancer. It's only after I'd spent a fruitless half hour unable to match any of my symptoms to those online that I would remember my lunch the day before where I had a salad with generous amounts of roasted beets.

I worried about going deaf and blind. I agonized about blood clots travelling from my calf to my heart. I fretted about a spate of headaches especially when, in my entire life, the number of headaches I have had can be counted on both hands. If I sneezed or coughed, I was concerned that I might throw out my back or dislocate my shoulder, as happened to a good friend of mine a few days after she turned 45.

When I finished mentally scrolling the list of ailments from which I might die, I would transfer all that anxiety and fear to my husband's mortality. I would run through the same list and imagine his death from any of these scenarios and add a few more: being crushed by a rogue front-end loader on a construction site, getting buried alive in a building collapse, or being involved in a car accident as he drove to work at 4:30 on a dark, snowy winter morning.

The anxiety was on replay all night long. Try as I might, I couldn't silence the beast. I tossed and turned. Occasionally, I would actually feel tears start to fall when I thought about life without my husband. Earlier that same day at dinner, I wanted him to choke on the butter-soaked corn on the cob he was slurping and chomping.

At 3:57 a.m., the dog came into the room, tail wagging. She had clearly heard my weeping/restlessness/moans of frustration and calculated in her canine mind that I needed some comfort. She jumped onto the bed, finding her place right alongside my sweaty body. She's an 85-pound dog, so when she shimmied her way closer to me, she pulled the comforter with her. I had a warm, cuddly dog on one side and an exposed, cold leg, hip, and upper arm on the other. In four minutes, I'd want to pull the cover back over me, but if I did that, the dog would growl, waking my husband, and my nighttime anxiety would be exacerbated by guilt that I woke him up 44 minutes before his alarm went off.

So I dealt with it and pet the dog, taking comfort in her soft fur and loving her so much for knowing exactly when I needed her. I lifted my head off my pillow and peeked at her adorable face. Her nose was nestled in the comforter, nuzzling my upper abdominal jelly roll. From this vantage point, I could see the white fur creeping over her face. She was eight years old, a senior by dog standards. I closed my eyes, and continued petting her, letting my hand settle on the scruff at the back of her neck. In the midst of that satisfying connection, I started to feel sadness. I was imagining life without our beloved dog. How many years of quality life did she have left? If she got really sick, would we opt for treatment or end her suffering? Why was I even thinking about this? It's the menopausal mind, set to autoplay.

On a different night, I lay in bed listening to the rain. A major storm moved into the area and a clap of thunder shook the house and woke my husband and I. The boys, now teenagers, did not stir. As the fat drops hammered the roof, I started panicking about money. We knew the roof was going to have to be replaced, but we were not ready for it. I wondered if the basement was flooding. I worried the DRICORE sub-flooring we installed when we renovated would fail. If it did its job, any water that found its way into the basement would drain under the flooring and leave our carpets and walls undamaged. But what if the water was at higher ground and started running down the walls from the first floor? The worry wormed into my brain and wouldn't let go. Our bank account was not flush, we didn't have significant savings or a rainy day fund. If shit went sideways, we were screwed. And broke.

As the rain eased up, my mind inevitably turned to my business. I thought about where I wanted to take it, how I could bring in more revenue, whether or not I was still in love with what I did every day. I worried about my inadequacies. I reflected on the great clients I have had over the years. I freaked out when I thought about all the things I might have forgotten: emails I didn't answer, bills I forgot to pay, projects I sent out into the world that were unfinished. The business voice in my head was messing with me, whispering cruelly that I had forgotten to add footage to a video, or that I had sent a client the wrong blog. I lay in bed, attempting to convince myself that there was nothing I could do about this at 2 a.m. and I would check things in the morning. Except I don't. That asshole who is living rent-free in my cerebrum manipulated me into getting out of bed and heading downstairs to my home office. I fired up the computer and checked everything, discovered I didn't colossally screw up and went back to bed, hoping I had quieted the anxiety enough to get some sleep.

But it doesn't take long for the next anxiety-driven symptom to show up. Without warning, my heart starts palpitating. It's pounding inside my chest with an irregular rhythm. I run through the mental checklist of the other signs of heart attack: jaw pain, arm pain, indigestion, difficulty breathing. I think maybe I feel some pain in my left jaw, but as soon as I focus on it, it disappears. I have no other issues other than indigestion, which is almost chronic at this stage in life. It's purely a menopausal coincidence that the spicy hot and sour soup I had at dinner has decided *now* is the time to reassert itself. The palpitations don't last long, just long enough to make me circle back to item number one on my mortality checklist: heart attack. As an obese, middle-aged woman whose activity level is slightly less than moderate and sometimes close to sloth-like, it's a valid concern. As I lie in bed, staring at the popcorn ceiling, I make promises to myself that I know I won't keep the minute a plate of crispy, salty bacon is in front of me.

You'd think all this thinking and planning and worrying would exhaust me. It does, but that doesn't mean I am going to sleep anytime soon. I turn over onto my left side and look at my husband's outline underneath the covers. I hold my breath, waiting for the rise of his chest. I cannot imagine life without him.

Breathe, damnit.

Jeff has mild sleep apnea, and tonight he has decided to forego his CPAP machine. Without the machine, he will stop breathing many times during the night. It can be fatal if left untreated, not just for the sufferer, but for the 50-something spouse lying next to him in bed hoping that she did not miss his last breath.

Breathe, damnit.

I wait, taking small, short breaths of my own, and pray.

Breathe, damnit.

Just as I am about to reach over and wake him, the characteristic gasp and gurgle erupts from his mouth and he takes a breath.

Phew.

He will not die tonight.

He will live another day to do something that irrationally annoys the fuck out of me.

TWENTY

THE SHAPE OF A POOP

C'mon Dana. You're really going to write a whole chapter on what happens in the guts? Yes, my lovelies, I am. The bowels, like the vagina, are one of those body parts that we never talk about freely. Pooping and farting is something everyone does, regardless of age, sex, or species, yet it is still somewhat of a taboo subject. We'll freely talk about our sex lives with our girlfriends. We'll share our labour stories. Over a glass of Chardonnay we'll laugh about the things we never thought we'd say in public ("Let go of your brother's penis!"). But the subject of how we poop, with what frequency, and when there might be a problem are things that we categorize under "Topics that Make us Uncomfortable." In fact, I may have started writing this chapter while my best friend disappeared for 30 minutes to the bathroom. I know what she's doing, but when she comes out, I'll pretend that I don't.

Metabolism is something that has plagued me my entire life. I've never had a strong and fast metabolism. I was born to hold on to popcorn for three days after ingestion. I spent too much time in my teen years trying to find ways to make my metabolism work faster, but it wasn't until I was almost 30 that I discovered my problem wasn't how my body processed food, but what I was putting into my mouth that was an issue. This was a pattern that was to be repeated during my perimenopausal journey.

I was frustrated by my inability to drop any weight. No matter how many salads I ate, or how few, the numbers on the scale crept up. I hired a personal trainer who essentially fired me after three months because my weight and my measurements were still the same.

"But I feel great," I told her. It was true. I was feeling strong and I was walking with my back straight and my boobs out. I had less stiffness when I woke in the morning. I was craving apples, for heaven's sake.

"Maybe once a week is not enough," she suggested.

"Okay," I nodded, "I think I can afford twice weekly." I paused, doing a quick mental calculation of what I would cut from the budget to make this happen. "You know what? I'll make it work." An image of a stronger, leaner me flashed across my mind. *Maybe this time it'll work...*

"Yeah, umm, except I can't," my trainer said. "I'm fully booked. Besides, my husband says maybe we're not the right fit and I can't expect all my clients to experience a transformation."

My eyes burned, but I managed to hold back the tears.

This bitch has never worked with a woman going through menopause. She's used to young clients who see changes in 20 minutes, not a 45-year-old, plus-sized chunk whose body needs six months of lead time before it figures out what is happening.

Even as I was lost in my own thoughts, she continued to

explain why this wasn't working for her. I stopped listening, stepped off the resistance band that was stretched under my feet and walked out. I was going to have to figure this out another way.

If you do a Google search for "metabolism during menopause" you will be assaulted with a plethora of diet plans, hormone fixes, and weight-loss techniques. The language around a lot of this bothers me. This is not a battle to be won, a problem you can solve with determination, or something you can easily stop. The slowing down of metabolism during menopause happens to every woman. It cannot be avoided.

Once I acknowledged that my body was producing less estrogen of its own free will, my mindset around my growing middle changed. I was going to have to let things happen until I was post-menopausal. That didn't mean I was going to sit on the couch all day, eating a bag of chips (but yes, I do have those days every now and then). I didn't give up on exercise. I shifted the focus away from the numbers on the scale. As I approached 50, it became imperative that I work on reducing the pain in my shoulder from an old injury. I needed more strength, not fewer calories. When I could lift my arm above my head, squat without losing my balance, or carry a bag of water softener salt down to the basement, all without pain, I could claim victory. My metabolism could do what it needed to do in the meantime.

The changes to my bowel started during peri-menopause, but they were so subtle, I didn't immediately notice. At first, it was small inconveniences like heartburn after a hot cup of coffee. I dismissed this as my body forgetting how to process hot coffee because as a mom of two littles who were not yet in school, my coffee was typically tepid. Then green peppers started repeating on me and if I ate one, either raw or cooked, I would spend the rest of the day apologizing for my grassy burps. Onions did the same, but with the added bonus of farts that felt like they burned my nose. As I progressed through perimenopause, my food intolerances and bowel changes got worse. Sushi caused horrible gastro-intestinal pain and I always vomited about 20 minutes after eating. That made for a very awkward meeting with a potential new client who insisted on taking me to lunch at his favourite sushi place. Instead of speaking up like a big girl and being honest about my physical inability to eat raw fish, I timed my ingestion in such a way so that I could get through the business deal, eat so as not to offend, and throw up 10 minutes after our lunch was over and we parted ways. It was worth it; I got the gig.

My intestinal issues were not limited to discomfort after eating. All sorts of new gurgles and gassiness made themselves known. My guts could rumble with gas so loudly that my husband thought maybe a train was passing nearby. Thankfully we were more than a decade into our marriage, long past the point of having to be polite about farting, because I could pass gas that rivalled the methane-producing flatulence of a cow. I didn't need beans or cabbage to prove my bowels were working. Chicken soup, toast with peanut butter, or a grilled cheese sandwich were equally suspect. In an attempt to quiet the noise and reduce the discomfort, I switched to decaffeinated coffee and started drinking herbal tea. After three miserable caffeine-free days, I decided I would rather burp and fart and enjoy my intestinal symphony than do without the boost.

When I poop also underwent some significant changes. Before perimenopause, I never paid attention to when I emptied my bowels, but suddenly, it became very relevant. Where I once was a get-out-of-bed-brush-my-teeth-and-poop girl, I was now a different woman, one who could shower, brush her teeth, have coffee and breakfast, and then poop. This change became apparent to me one morning when I was heading out of the house for work, having done all those things, except I gave my guts extra time to work. I was fortunate that I was only about a kilometre from my house when my bowels felt the immediate need to empty. I turned around and went home, laughing to myself as I sat on the toilet. Mom was right. I should have gone before I left the house.

The digestive tract will never be the same once you start perimenopause. I suffered from constipation and diarrhea and lived in a general state of indigestion. I felt like I was reliving my second pregnancy. Periodically, I had mystery abdominal cramps that started on the right side of my abdomen and moved to my left, like a food baby that was working its way through my intestines.

Over the course of six years, my medicine cabinet underwent a transformation. The children's Advil, cough syrup, and Benadryl were pushed to the back to make room for the new range of medicines and supplements: Senokot (a natural laxative), Metamucil, and warehouse-club sized bottles of Tums. I always had a roll of Rolaids in my purse. The antacids were such a vital part of my life that I was painfully (literally) aware when Rolaids, Pepcid, and Tums were each recalled and pulled from the shelves. Thankfully, this didn't happen all at the same time.

The shape of my poop was another topic that held great interest for me. I would check after every movement to visually evaluate the shape and consistency. I paid close attention to what my food input did to my poop output. To the horror of my husband and our two sons, I was compelled to share this information with them. At the dinner table. I'm sure my boys would have preferred I give them the sex talk every evening rather than share my bowel movement history.

TWENTY-ONE

THE WOMAN OF YOUR DREAMS

I want to prepare you for the crazy ride of the nighttime pictures that will play out in your head and stay with you for the whole day. As I was progressing through perimenopause, my dreams became more emotionally charged and more vivid.

Just this week, I woke from a dream I could barely remember. I know something happened that either broke my heart or left me extremely disappointed, but I can't recall exactly what. After I woke, just before 5 a.m., I carried the wisps of this dream with me into the shower. Instead of clearing with the steam, the dream leftovers festered like an infected sore. By the time I was dressed and ready for the day, I was pissed off. The betrayal from my dream infused itself into my whole being. I was in a crappy mood for the rest of the day over something that never happened.

This is a phenomenon common to menopausal women. As hormones shift and progesterone and estrogen levels decrease, we spend less time in REM (rapid eye movement) sleep. It's in REM sleep where we experience our most vivid dreams. Before the hormonal havoc of menopause, we stay asleep longer and this is why we don't tend to remember the dreams. But during the menopausal journey, we spend less time in deep sleep. The more we wake up, the more likely we are to remember the REM dreams.

One woman I know had a variation of dreams about being pregnant. Sometimes, she would deliver the baby without even knowing she was pregnant and would panic about not being prepared with supplies or furniture. When she woke, the panic was still with her and left her feeling lost for the rest of the day.

My favourite is from my friend, Paula, who dreamt that her husband was cheating on her. In her words: "It's not so much the cheating that gets me, it's his blasé attitude to it in the dreams. He always says he's leaving me. When I wake up, I slug him for cheating and then I stay mad the entire day because the dreams are so real."

My dreams during perimenopause and beyond were vivid, with colours so bright I felt like I was in a movie. The human interactions were so real and fluid. Conversations happened exactly as they would in real life, with interruptions and emotions. My dreams were populated by people I knew and complete strangers. I travelled the world, ate decadent meals, and won marathons. That last one was my favourite. I was the only person on the planet who, at 295 pounds, ran a full marathon and was the first to cross the finish line. I barely broke a sweat and earned a sponsorship contract with a major athletic brand. I woke up feeling that victory and it followed me for the whole day. I was a champion. Nothing could stop me if I set my mind to it. My real-world self rewarded my dream-world self with a justified caloric binge of a fried chicken sandwich and French fries.

On the other side of the feel-good, but highly unlikely,

dreams are the ones that leave me heartbroken and devastated. These dreams really shake me and I think about them all day. The worst part is these dreams are usually recurring and have plagued me for years. One dream involves a work colleague who befriends me, asks me to mentor her, and then steals my business out from under me. In another dream, my ex-husband comes back to me to beg forgiveness and after I take him back and we live happily for a few years, I discover he has been living a double life as a gay man with a whole second family. I wake feeling angry, stupid, and betrayed. That is not a good day.

I've also experienced dreams where nothing made sense. We've all had dreams like this, whether we are menopausal or not. The difference to me was I carried my mood swings, irrationality, and sense of humour into this dream world. In one dream, I meet a chiselled hunk of a man. He falls in love with me and asks me to marry him. I consent, but only if I can stroke his abs whenever and wherever I choose. I am not in love with him at all. He is a trophy, Rodin's *Thinker* in the flesh. He consents and I become a weirdo who caresses his abdomen like I'm petting a dog. No one else seems to notice this odd behaviour. And then he ghosts me. I don't panic, I don't send a million texts, I don't feel heartbroken. Instead of feeling the loss, I go swimming. I swim laps like an athlete in training. I wake up during an underwater flip at the wall. I swear I can smell chlorine.

During this stage in my life, as my libido was snuffing itself out, my sexy dreams inexplicably became almost pornographic. Even though I was asleep, I felt my body react to every touch, caress, and kiss. I was sexually alive in my dreams, more so than I was at any time in my real life. I wasn't overly promiscuous in the dreams, I just had really great sex. Every single encounter, whether relationship-based or a one-night stand, had a happy ending. My body was a temple to whoever was worshipping me in that particular dream. I was revered as a voluptuous and curvy goddess, admired as an athletic and compelling icon, and loved for being smart and witty. Everything was perfect. My climax in my dream was powerful enough to wake me, breathless and feeling every nerve in my body come alive.

I would quickly close my eyes again, trying to slip back into that bliss. I tried to put myself back into the exact place where I awoke. The story was still there, waiting for me to write it however I chose. I would smile to myself, feeling the edges of sleep wrapping its pillowy arms around me again. I was ready to finish what had been started. Then the voice of reason would interrupt me, reminding me I had a husband right next to me who would be willing to help me continue my ecstasy. I don't wake him though. If I woke Jeff, I'd have to explain why I'm waking him, assure him I am, in fact, coming on to him, and wait for him to make a trip to the bathroom before we started at square one.

I want to go back to the dream where the foreplay was already done and I was lost in the throes of passion. The things I could do in my dreams — the way I could move my body — could not be replicated in real life. So, yeah, I just wanted to roll over and go back to sleep, back into the ethereal world of perfect, exciting, climactic sex.

It's not to be, though. Seconds after I have closed my eyes and mentally rewound to the point in my dream where I woke up, my bladder has other plans.

TWENTY-TWO

VITAMINS AND MINERALS

Being a women is expensive, but being a woman with menopause can drain your bank account via supplements, miracle creams, and rocks. During my last year of perimenopause when I was halfway through my year without a period, I began searching for ways to feel better. I was done with being tired all the time. I wanted better gut health, better sleep, and better moods. I was looking for clarity of the mind, a deeper sense of purpose, and affirmation that I was going to be okay. Naturally, I turned to rocks.

For the next six months, I was enamoured with crystals. Every day, I made intentional choices for which beaded bracelets would be wrapped around my wrist. If I needed to release some anxiety, I wore tiger's eye. My choice for a networking event was hematite, to ward off any negativity either from myself or others. My moonstone mala hung from my neck whenever I was searching for hope and abundance. I put a reddish-orange carnelian stone in my pocket to boost my confidence when I had to present before a group. I dropped a heart-shaped rose quartz into my bra before I went to a meeting with a potential new client because I wanted them to love me.

I found myself rubbing a stone when I needed peace of mind. I learned all about grounding and shunned my shoes in favour of walking barefoot on gravel. I don't know if I got any closer to the planet, but my feet were certainly better exfoliated. I paid attention to the moon cycles so I could recharge and clean my crystals. Once every month, the patio table in the backyard resembled a cluttered discount table at a community hall garage sale. My kids rolled their eyes at me and Jeff tolerated my newfound love for all things rocks.

I wore out the bracelets, so much so, that during a presentation I was giving, my energetic hand-waving caused one of my bracelets to snap apart and send tiger's eye beads flying. They soared across the carpet, under chairs, and even into the cheek of one of the attendees. Instead of being mortified, I laughed and shared that this was sign from the universe for me to get some new bracelets.

I met some fascinating people who were deeply entrenched in the spiritual world. I worked with clients who were angel healers, reiki masters, and intuitive leaders. I was introduced to men and women who had found inner peace and were genuinely invested in helping me find mine. I tried to fully absorb everything I was learning, but I always felt like I was on the margins. It wasn't because I didn't believe, it was just that I was proceeding with caution. I couldn't quite understand how a $600 crystal necklace could help you fix your intimacy with your partner. My logical brain piped in with its opinion that the money might be better spent on some couple's therapy. I know for certain that if I came home with a walnut-sized lapis lazuli and told my husband it would make our relationship more meaningful, he would very likely walk out the door and find a hotel to stay in for a week for less than I spent on a crystal dream. And it would have a deeper effect on our relationship. I drew the line at extravagant spending, but I became acutely aware that for some there is no price too high to pay for believing in something. Fortunately for me, and my marriage, the rocks lost their lustre and became background decor and fun baubles.

๛

My next venture was into the world of herbs with a particular focus on sage. I had heard from many sources in my new circle that burning sage in my house was a great way to get rid of a variety of issues that might be plaguing me. I smudged my entire house, from the basement to the master bedroom, hoping to rid our home of unwanted spirits, negative energy, tainted molecules, dormant viruses, and obstacles to sleep quality. My whole heart was in this. I made sure to get into every corner, waving my cluster of burning herbs around like a grandma with a feather duster. My grandmother would have been horrified that I was burning dried leaves inside the house and leaving trails of ash everywhere. She would have thought I was crazy and told me to go to school to "be something."

By the time I made it to the second floor of the house, I was on my third bunch of sage. Instead of holding the raw bunch of leaves in my hand, I had it sitting inside a mug, the smoke wafting out like steam from a coffee. When I was done, my whole house smelled like I had hosted a marijuana party and then tried to cover up the smell with cedar. I performed this ritual while Jeff was travelling, since I knew he would either

a) make fun of me

b) send me out to buy some Reactine to calm his allergies

c) find somewhere else to be that didn't smell like a frat house, or worst of all

d) open all the windows to air out the house, thus negating all my effort to spiritually cleanse all of us.

When the kids came home from school, my eldest didn't even ask, he just knowingly rolled his eyes. My younger son wrinkled his nose and blurted out "WHAT IS THAT STINK?" and waved his hand in front of his nose. He was the more sensitive of our children, so I explained to him what I had done and why.

"I smudged the house with sage to clear out any negative energy. I know it's smelly, but it will help align our chakras."

"I don't know what that means, but okay. You do you, Mom."

I still had some sage left and I packed it away in the kitchen cupboard. It sat there, unused, for another year and a half before I threw it out. My husband had started cooking meals for us and I was worried he would use it in a beef stew, resulting in a kind of cleansing none of us would appreciate. I can't say conclusively whether the sage was effective, but at least it was more affordable than lapis lazuli.

❦

When I was out of my mystic phase, I moved into the more commonly accepted realm of vitamins. I spent more time than I'd like to admit standing in the herbal medicine aisle of the drugstore, phone in hand, looking up the various supplements and their uses. I started with the simple things like vitamin B complex, hoping to boost my red blood cell growth, clear up my digestive issues, and clear my brain fog. I can't definitively say I saw any benefits from that, but I can confirm my pee turned bright yellow.

I moved on to omega-3 to combat my palpitating heart, but I couldn't tolerate the bad breath and excess gas. If I had to be farting, I'd rather it be caused by drinking coffee. I'm not sure why I expected anything less from fish oil. I discovered black cohosh, which promised to alleviate hot flashes, night sweats, and insomnia. I later laid in bed watching the hours pass, dripping wet and stewing over how much I spent on that bottle. I was already familiar with melatonin for helping me fall asleep, but that wasn't ever a problem for me. Staying asleep was the issue. I looked at valerian root and chamomile and an online search took me someplace unexpected: a tea shop.

As a person who enjoys a warm cup of tea in the evening, this seemed to be the perfect solution. I could fulfill my nighttime ritual and reap the benefits of helpful herbs mixed with decadent flavours like caramel and coconut. During this period, I switched from black tea to rooibos and found a vast assortment of teas to please my palate while calming my mind. It worked for a while until I got bored with the same flavours and realized my premium tea habit was forcing us to sacrifice some of the things we loved as a family, like regular groceries.

This period of searching for answers lasted for about two and a half years, beyond perimenopause and into post-menopause. I did not consult my doctor, but not because I didn't want to. Despite the rampage of symptoms, it never occurred to me during my seven-year journey through menopause to seek professional medical help. I didn't consider that maybe medication was what I needed, I was just trying to get through my days with my sanity intact. I don't regret anything I tried and I didn't go so far over the edge of rational thought that I did anything foolish. It was a season in my menopausal life that I wanted to explore. When we look for answers to what ails us, we have to be willing to step out of our comfort zones. It's what we find in our fear that makes us stronger.

TWENTY-THREE

THIS IS YOUR MID-LIFE CRISIS CALLING

There has never been a lot of attention paid to the mid-life crisis in women, simply because the focus was always on men. How could it not be? It's a world filled with clichés we are all too familiar with.

As men hit this stage, they pine for their youth. You can see it in the men who chase younger women or wear expensive designer jeans or pull their vinyl out of the attic. Men in mid-life are sneered at for buying that convertible sports car they always wanted, for completely sucking at sneaking around with someone other than their wife, or for whining about how much they hate their top-level, well-compensated executive position at work. There's a restlessness that comes with a man's mid-life crisis. They are dissatisfied with work, with the rut of daily life, with the passage of time.

As much as I'd like to man-bash and say they need to get over that shit, I can't. Women in mid-life are really not much better. It's a cruel intention of nature that our mid-life and our menopause occur roughly at the same time. Now,

I'm no expert on this topic, but I am a writer, so I observe things that most people miss. I think about things that are ridiculous, as my Google search history will attest to, and sometimes I share those thoughts out loud. Or in a book.

I've noticed a few trends among the women in my world that I suspect are driven by the hormonal changes combined with passing the age of 40. I don't have any proof that I am right about any of this, but if I see something happening and it's repeated, that's a trend.

Marriages are ending with the suddenness of a tsunami. Several of my friends have up and left their husbands, moved out, and decided it was time to be happy. Every time this happens, it catches me off-guard because I thought she *was* happy. We were at their house for dinner last month and we had a fabulous time. There was no hint of tension. We got happy-drunk, ate more than we should have, and laughed at life. I suspect the husband was just as shocked as I was when the wife told him the marriage was over, and oh, yeah, because she spent the last 18 years raising the kids she needed to live in the basement until she landed on her feet.

Some of my more assertive friends sent their soon-to-be ex-husbands to the basement with a bar fridge and a hot plate and wished him the best of luck. A few of my more financially stable friends were able to move out into their own basement apartment in someone else's house. They were on a new path to happiness and independence and it didn't matter if there were millipedes crawling under the washing machine. They were free. They had left a marriage that left them feeling unloved and suffocated. "People change," they said. Except they don't. What changed was what they were willing to settle for. They woke up one morning, looked around the house and home they built for the past 10 or 15 or 20 years and wanted to take a match to the whole thing.

A mid-life crisis isn't the same as menopause; it's a sudden awareness of what your life is. In the space of three years, at least a dozen of my friends and acquaintances dissolved their marriages. Not one to pry, I never asked for any details, but occasionally over coffee, they would tell me the story. There were the usual culprits and some surprising revelations: growing apart, infidelity, hidden drug addictions, and a strong desire to engage in a swinger lifestyle. Some of my friends told me they realized that they never really loved their husbands, or that they grew to see they had nothing in common once the kids were gone.

When I brought up the idea that menopause could cloud our judgment, almost every single woman told me that it was exactly the opposite. The mind muddle of menopause made them see what they had previously turned a blind eye to. One friend shrugged her shoulders, conceding maybe I was right, but she was still happy to have left. Menopause just gave her the courage to say "Fuck this" and leave. That's the part of menopause that feels really good, that spark and sense of fearlessness that propels you to action. It's that same feeling that pushed her to join a gym and shed tons of weight. That feeling of elation is what drive others to find a tattoo parlour and begin inking like they are in a motorcycle club.

While motorcycles are on your mind, I'd like to point out that no fewer than a dozen of my friends decided in their mid-to-late forties to take bike lessons. Like men with their sport cars, women in middle age are searching for an adrenalin rush and want to be out on the open road with something stable and strong and steely between their legs.

My friends on bikes have opened my eyes to a whole world I didn't know existed, one in which women ride and race together. I've never once been on a motorcycle, so I can't pretend to understand what it feels like. I have zero interest in driving at high speed on two wheels without doors. I like the safety of my SUV and if I want a thrill, I'll open up the sunroof and let my hair get messy in the rush of air.

Another trend I am watching from the sidelines revolves around tattoos. I've lost count of how many of my perimenopausal, newly divorced friends have added ink to their bodies. One went from zero tattoos to four in less than a year. I've been shown tattoos that are simply words and ones of symbols that hold special meaning for their hosts. A friend started her artwork on her shoulder and I watched as it grew into a full sleeve over a couple of years. Regardless of the size or location, the tattoos all have one thing in common. They are markers of an event or a transition in life.

Way back when I was a newspaper reporter, I wrote a two-page feature story on tattoos (think: luxurious read on a Sunday morning). At the time, I thought tattoos were part of a subculture and that only people of a certain demographic (think: bikes and prison) would subject themselves to that kind of pain. Of course, you already know how wrong I was on that one. I spent weeks researching and visiting tattoo parlours and interviewing all kinds of people. By the time the story was written, I had a new appreciation of the art form and a better understanding of why people feel driven to have permanent ink injected into their skin. It's not something I would do to myself, but I can gaze at a woman's upper arm like I'm lost in van Gogh's *Starry Night*.

Among all the new furniture, bikes, and tats, I see

women who are happy and fulfilled, even as their bodies betray them. They fight like hell every day — to raise their kids on their own, to embrace a new direction they never saw coming, to dance like a fiend on TikTok — even though they are tired, bloated, and suddenly craving a corn dog.

TWENTY-FOUR

THE POST-IT NOTE

We need to stop framing menopause as a disappointing loss. There is no question this stage of our lives is filled with upheaval and chaos, but a woman's life is never black and white anyways. Ask any (brave and slightly drunk) man and he will tell you that women are complex. Ask a (smart) married man, and he'll respond with "Yes, dear" to whatever you say. Women's bodies are built tough. We can handle the worst pain of childbirth and provide the best comfort a soft body can offer. We are pillows to our children and edgy leaders to our employees. We know how to apologize when we are wrong (especially if we are Canadian) and champion ourselves when we are right.

A friend suggested that menopause be renamed "menostop" in reference to our periods stopping. The more I thought about it and as I was writing about it, it became clear that this stage, for me, was a really big pause. For seven years, I was suspended between who I was working to become and who I really am. I like to think of this journey as a rest stop along the road of trying to break through the glass ceiling or to be a better mom than the one I had. I can use this time to figure out how life works and examine the new road that stretches ahead of me after I've figured out who I am, what I want to do and what brings me joy. Meno*stop* is a dead end; meno*pause* is chance to sit back and map out a more fulfilling route.

I'm not trying to start a revolution. I'm not calling for women to hit the streets with placards announcing the #MenopauseMovement. I am inviting you to accept this stage of life and run with it. Don't fight what you cannot change even as the changes are raging inside and outside your skin. Embrace what is happening.

Now that I am post-menopausal, I wish that early in my stages of crazy someone would have told me what I recently told a friend of mine who was diagnosed with cancer.

Put a post-it note on your bathroom mirror with these words on it: "Not today, motherfucker."

These three words can be a call to action just as much as they can give you permission to have a shitty day. It's a mantra I could have applied to every mood swing and frustration. I could have felt the power of these words as I examined the insomnia-induced bags under my eyes and pulled out my concealer. I could have looked at my bathroom scale and said, "Not today, motherfucker."

The range of change is so different for every woman and this book just tells my own tale. You may be emotionally all over the map or you may be limited to one emotion (rage seems to top the list). Your metabolism can become slower than a toddler getting dressed to leave the house or it can speed up so much that you barely finish swallowing when you have to race to the bathroom. Your mind may be filled with noise and chaos or you may find yourself standing in a backyard shed with no idea of when your husband bought and built it. You can experience none of these things or all of these things. There is no reasoning with your hormones and no controlling the outcome. Even with medications, things will go awry.

Hang in there, my sisters. There is hope. I emerged into my post-menopausal world with blazing hot confidence. By the time my hormones were settled and my eggs were long gone, I felt comfortable with *all* of myself for the first time in my life. I know who I am, what my gifts are, and what place I hold in the world (the evidence is this book). A lot of days I feel like I can skip through life not giving a damn what you think. I'll think about tossing glitter in the air, but I won't, because I don't want that shit everywhere. I'll listen to what someone has to say and zip my lips. I don't have to say anything, but I take comfort in knowing the option is there for me. If I piss you off and you never speak to me again, it's okay. I might be the asshole you no longer want in your life.

I've got a solid relationship with my husband and eventually he'll be done slurping his soup and I can love him again. My teenage boys hide behind the closed doors of their bedrooms and I have no problem with that. I'm not worried about them watching porn (which they are) or that they talk shit with their friends online as they shoot things or each other. I have made sure our boys know that neither of those things are real life. I am grateful that I know where they are, even if I'm not completely sure I know what they are doing. I've given them as much information about menopause as I can ("Mom is pissed off, but not at you. You're just in the line of fire."), hoping they will remember this when the women in their lives hit this stage.

When you emerge from your years of transition, things will never be the same. You may have a new wardrobe. You might discover you are a morning person after all. You'll be okay with having cold leftover tuna casserole for breakfast or frying the homemade soppressata your friend gave you because you don't have any bacon and you want something salty and crispy. You'll develop new skills, like sourcing and plucking your chin hairs without needing a mirror. You'll feel decadent about making coffee at 3 a.m. and settling onto the couch to get lost in a book. You'll nap later. You'll adjust to this new life and you'll be thrilled about what the next 50 years will bring you (I likely will not write a book about that, though).

So go ahead and create your own post-it note. Hug your dog even though she licks your new reading glasses as you wrap your arms around her neck. Eat the cupcake. Buy a new lipstick and go for glossy if that's your jam. Wear those fabulous boots that make you feel like you can kick some ass. Be strong and embrace all the glory of getting this far. Your uterus has stepped down and it's now your time to show the world who you are and what you are capable of doing. But first, please go get your handbag and throw out that three-year-old tampon you've been holding on to, just in case. You're done now.

NOTES

2. Hormones

1. Name has been changed because we are no longer friends and I don't want an awkward conversation.

5. Periods

1. Name changed upon request. I don't blame her. That's a very disturbing event that belongs in a Stephen King novel.

ACKNOWLEDGMENTS

I owe a debt of gratitude to my beta readers who stepped up to help make this book better. Not only did they point out the areas that needed work, they were extremely candid in sharing their own experiences with menopause. Thank you to Carrie Paxson, Christine Tulk, Giuliana Melo, Heather Flanagan, Laura Ballerini, Melissa Neville, and Shandra Carlson for taking the time to read the early draft and give me some new things to think about.

I appreciate the women who answered the call for menopause stories and agreed to let me name them in these pages: Valery Klassen, Janis Doherty, and Yvonne Laanstra.

A big hug and thanks to Corlie Garanito, who despite telling me she is the worst beta reader ever, is actually one of the best cheerleaders a writer could hope to have in her circle of trust.

Thank you Jackie Appleby for supporting the idea of this project from the start.

Thank you to my editor, Zoey Duncan, who did such a stellar job with *The Girl in the Gold Bikini* that there was never any question who I would hire to edit this book. You are so good at what you do and a gift to any writer.

To Jeff, Mason, and Westin: in case the dedication wasn't enough, I need to tell you that without you my life would be so very different. While I dream about a carefree life of travel and fantastic boots and handbags, I know that you three fill my heart in ways shopping in Paris at Louis Vuitton never could.

ABOUT THE AUTHOR

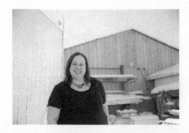

Dana Goldstein is an author of memoir and middle grade fiction. She is a natural born storyteller and has written for newspapers and magazines throughout North America. She currently lives in Calgary with her husband, two sons and a diva of a dog. Murder on my Mind is her second book.

Manufactured by Amazon.ca
Bolton, ON